The Slimming Foodie

IN MINUTES

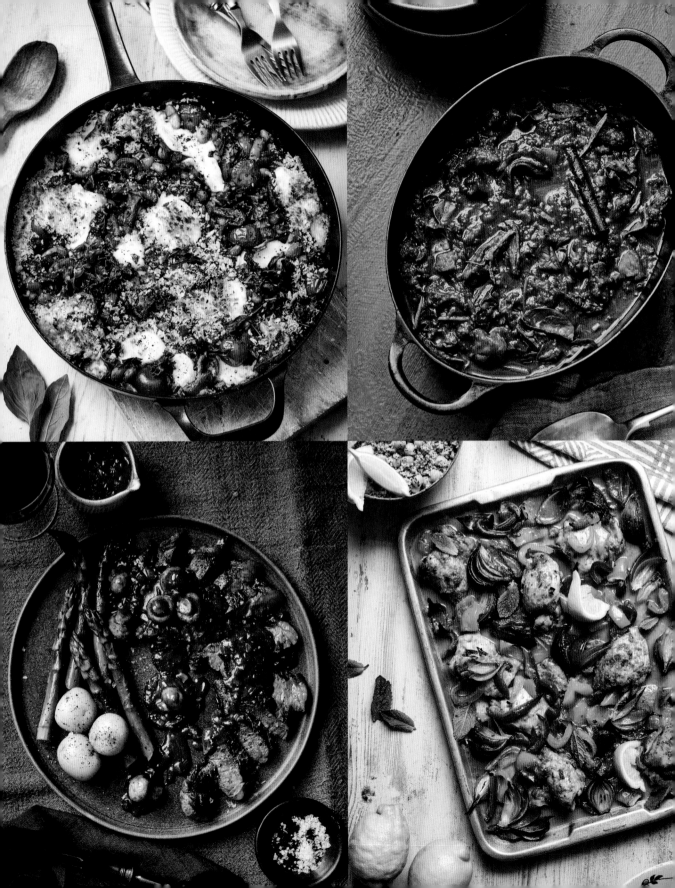

The Slimming Foodie

IN MINUTES

100+ QUICK-COOK RECIPES UNDER 600 CALORIES

PIP PAYNE

ASTER*

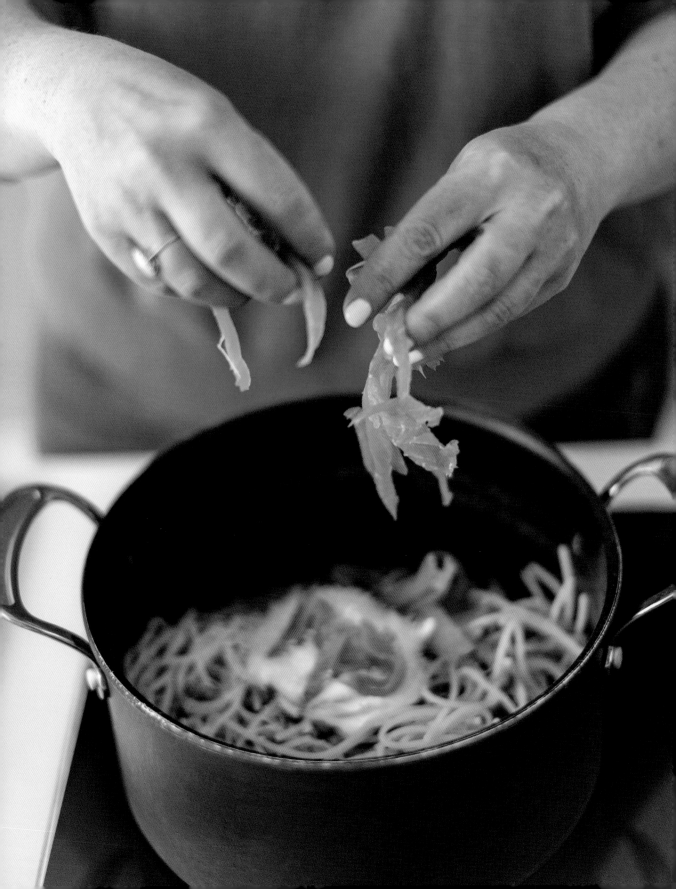

CONTENTS

INTRODUCTION

The Slimming Foodie has always been about making life in the kitchen as easy as possible when preparing healthy food, and, as a busy mum of two, I have spent years simplifying recipes and finding ways to cook delicious meals that aren't labour-intensive or fiddly.

Fresh, delicious meals don't have to take hours of your time, and this book is all about giving you varied meal options. They can all either be prepared and cooked in 30 minutes or less, or they are 'slam-dunk' dinners which can be prepared and thrown into one pot in 20 minutes or less, then left alone to slow-cook.

You will also find, dotted throughout the book, my **Three ways with...** sections. These explore the versatility of having a few key meal components – such as different varieties of pesto, say, or salsa – that can elevate the ingredients in your refrigerator to a new level. They will help you work with what you have, to create great food.

When you are keeping an eye on calories, you can't rely on fats to make the food taste good, as do many recipes you will find elsewhere. But I have a few key low-calorie tricks to secure fast flavour in minimal time, and these are the most important for this book:

- **Gather a few superstar ingredients**
  These can really do some of the hard work for us, providing fantastic 'ready-to-go' flavour to complement your dishes. Building a store cupboard with these key ingredients – such as sweet chilli sauce, gochujang paste, soy sauce and balsamic vinegar – will make cooking quick meals a complete breeze. I have tried to ensure that where a recipe requires a more unusual ingredient, it is used in at least one other recipe in the book to help you to use it up.

- **Always have dried herbs and spices to hand**
  They can be used in so many different ways to create an astounding variety of meals. Again, building up a store cupboard will make your cooking life a breeze.

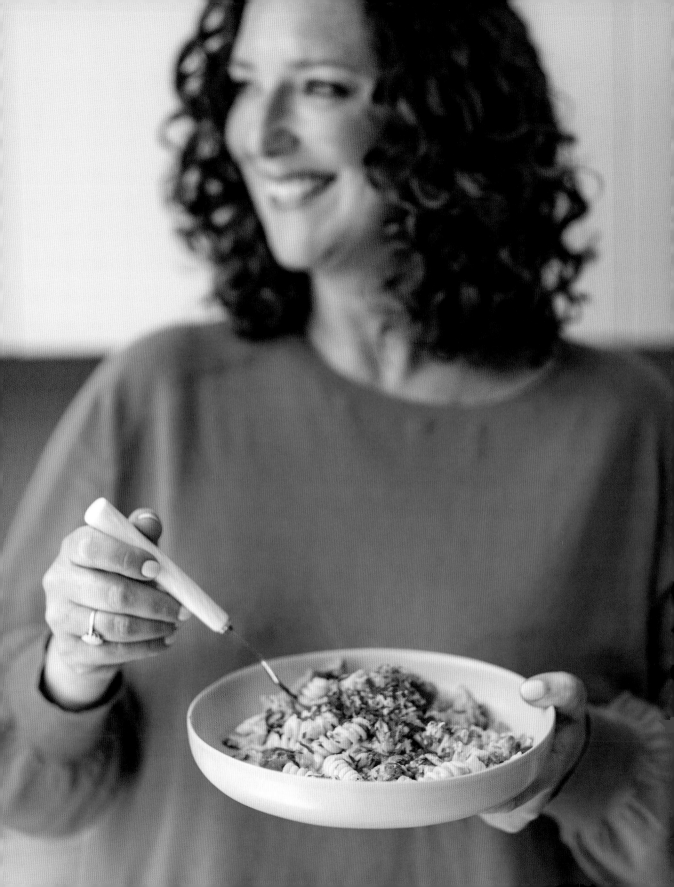

- **Know the power of fresh herbs**
  The huge variety available can add depth of flavour and fantastic fresh taste without any hassle at all, and if you have a few pots of your own at home (all you need is a windowsill!) they can always be on hand when you need them.

I hope that you love the recipes in this book. Please feel free to share photos and videos of your creations, tagging me, on social media… I love to see my food being brought to life!

KITCHEN KIT

Having the right kit will help you to take the hassle out of home cooking. The key items that will make this book easy to use and stay true to the prep times given are:

EQUIPMENT

- **Sauté pan with a lid**
  You will need a small variety of pans to cook these meals, but the sauté pan is by far my most used. It's perfect for frying, but you can build up a sauce in there too.

- **Good-quality sharp knife**
  Without this, chopping will be laboured and will slow everything up. Regularly sharpening your knife will keep it in peak chopping condition for many years.

- **Garlic crusher**
  Fresh garlic is such a key ingredient, but I find it can be a chore to finely chop it; a garlic crusher just makes this job quick and easy every time.

- **Microplane**
  Lemon, lime and orange zest can make a huge difference to a meal, and a Microplane will take a fine layer of zest off the fruit in seconds. A regular zester is fine, but will take longer and not produce such fine zest. I also find a Microplane the most efficient means to finely grate Parmesan cheese.

- **Measuring spoons**
  Generally, I have measured the amounts of dried herbs, spices, vinegars, sauces and so on by spoons, in order to give you a really accurate guide.

APPLIANCES

- **Stick blender**
  The quickest and easiest way to blend soups and sauces.

- **Food processor**
  This can save an awful lot of chopping, and many also have attachments for grating. You don't need an expensive model, a supermarket own-brand processor will do the job just fine.

- **Mini chopper**
  One of my most-used bits of kitchen kit, this is invaluable for making spice pastes and sauces in minutes, or for finely chopping smaller amounts of ingredients that might get lost in a bigger food processor. It's also much quicker to wash up than a larger food processor.

- **Meat thermometer**
  If you aren't confident about knowing when meat is cooked, then a meat thermometer can provide great peace of mind, as it accurately shows you when the meat has reached the required temperature. If in doubt, check it.

- **Slow-cooker**
  These are so handy and excellent for meals that take just moments to prepare, then you simply leave them to cook for hours. I use a 3.5-litre (6¼ pint) slow-cooker. All the recipes in my Slam-dunk Dinners chapter (see pages 168–187) use a slow-cooker.

GENERAL COOKING NOTES

- **Prep and cook times**
  I have personally tested all these recipes and written the prep and cooking times. I am a home cook, not a chef, so my chopping skills are very average, therefore I feel that the times I have estimated should be accurate as a guide for most people. I use a fan oven and keep a thermometer in it for every recipe I test, so the cook times are as accurate as I can make them. There are so many variables that can affect this, and all hobs and ovens will operate slightly differently. I have provided guidance and tips on how to judge whether the food is cooked in the recipes here, but remember that sometimes you may need to adjust the timings I give to suit your own appliances.

- **Ingredients**
  If you go to the index at the back of this book, you will find the names of ingredients and all the recipes that they are used in. So if, for example, you buy a big bag of kale for one recipe, look at the index and you will find some other ways of using it up in the book.

- **Oil**
  For most of my recipes I use a spray oil. I have a refillable food-grade spray bottle, and for most of these meals just a few sprays will be enough to do the necessary frying. Sometimes, though, you just need a little more than a spray, and then I might use a measured amount of butter or oil; this might be for flavour or just because the ingredients require a little more to cook properly. As the fats are always added in small amounts, when a meal is divided into portions they won't mean a big jump in calories, but may make a big difference to the flavour or to successful cooking. Of course, if you aren't watching the calorie content of meals, then using more oil or butter for frying won't ruin any of these recipes. I do also use low-calorie cooking spray occasionally; I find it particularly helpful for giving great coverage when cooking things in the oven.

- **Calories**
  The calorie counts stated in the recipes are for a single portion, and do not include serving suggestions or side dishes. Calorie calculations can vary based on the precision of measurements, the brand of ingredients (for example, cans of light coconut milk can vary greatly in calorie content), or the source of your nutritional data. The information provided here is intended as a guide.

- **Portion sizes**

  I work these out based on both personal experience and recommended portions. Of course, appetites and family set-ups can vary hugely, so you may need to adjust these to suit your own family. I often suggest side dishes, and cooking extra vegetables is always a good way to increase the size and filling power of a meal.

- **Freezing**

  I have made suggestions for which meals I think are freezer friendly and will reheat well. If you are freezing food, it's important to always let it cool fully before freezing it. I usually use airtight, washable plastic containers or freezer bags, and have learned to always label them with their contents and the date of freezing, to keep track. I have also found that keeping a 'freezer meal inventory' stuck to the refrigerator, writing on new additions and crossing out what has been used, helps me to use things up, rather than leave them languishing in the freezer for too long. Food should always be thoroughly defrosted before reheating; leaving it in the refrigerator overnight will allow it to defrost at a safe temperature.

HELPFUL TIP

Look out for these symbols at the top of each recipe page:

SUITABLE FOR VEGETARIANS

FREEZER FRIENDLY

CHAPTER GUIDE

Divided into eight chapters, I hope this book will give you a quick and easy solution when hunger strikes:

BREAKFAST & BRUNCH
Some quick ideas to help you make a delicious, filling morning meal.

MEAT-FREE DAYS
As many of us become more aware of our meat consumption and the importance of eating more vegetables, I've given some great plant-centred ideas.

MIDWEEK WINNERS
Whether you're dashing to the supermarket to pick up something easy, or raiding the cupboards to rustle something up, I've created some easy ideas for tasty midweek wins.

FAMILY FAVOURITES
It's important to be able to eat as a family, without having to cook everyone separate meals. With two quite fussy eaters of my own, I am well aware of common texture and taste dislikes in kids. I have shared some ideas that have worked well for my own family, as well as ingredient swaps that might work for yours.

FAKEAWAYS
A weekend takeaway can have a big effect on our weekly calorie intake, so being able to make takeaway-style meals or special dinners at home can only be a good thing. Some of these are slightly more indulgent than others, but still allow you to maintain a healthy balance.

SLAM-DUNK DINNERS
Meals that can be thrown into the slow-cooker in 20 minutes or less and left alone to cook, while you get on with your day.

SNACKS & SIDES
Quick dips, snacks and sides to fill a hole, satisfy a craving (healthily!), or get everyone keen to eat their greens.

SWEET TOOTH
Everyone needs to allow themselves the occasional treat, and being able to share a slice of cake with friends, or bake with your kids, is invaluable. These are healthier ideas for bakes and desserts that still taste great.

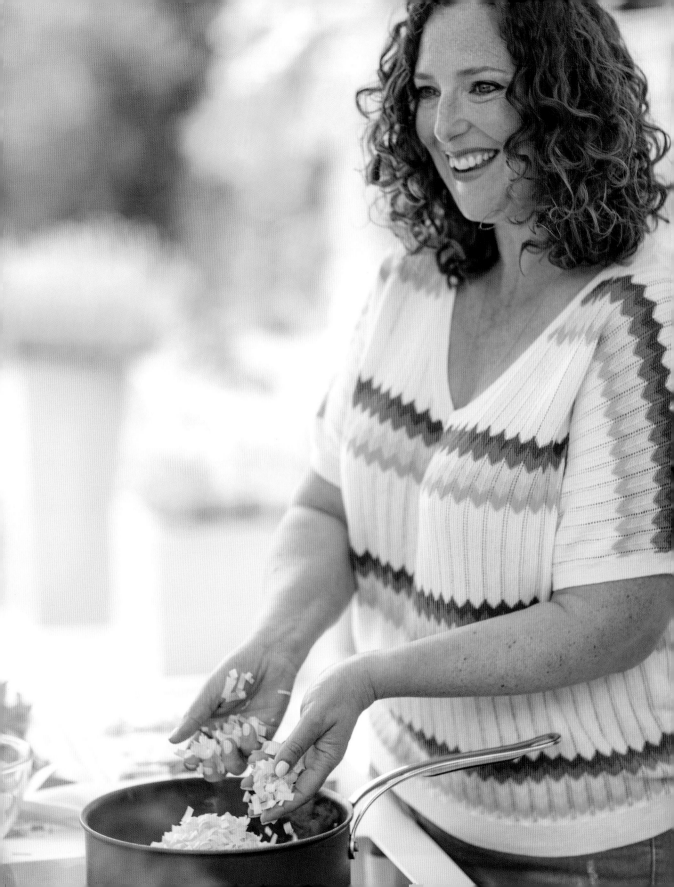

CHAPTER 1

BREAKFAST & BRUNCH

HOB GRANOLA

I've only started eating granola in the past couple of years and it's not always easy to find one that is low in sugar. Homemade just tastes so much better. My favourite things in granola are the nuts and seeds, and toasting them as I do in this recipe makes them taste amazing! If you make a small batch like this it can cover breakfasts for a week; I have it either with yogurt and fresh fruit, or as a topping for porridge.

PREP TIME: 5 MINUTES
COOK TIME: 6 MINUTES

2 tablespoons pure maple syrup
1 teaspoon vanilla extract
80g (2¾oz) jumbo oats
20g (¾oz) flaked almonds
1 tablespoon pumpkin seeds
1 tablespoon sunflower seeds
2 tablespoons chia seeds
¼ teaspoon salt
¼ teaspoon ground cinnamon

1. In a small bowl, mix together the maple syrup and vanilla extract.
2. In a large frying pan, dry-fry the oats over a medium heat for 3 minutes, stirring every now and again.
3. Push the oats to one side and add the almonds, pumpkin seeds, sunflower seeds and chia seeds. Dry-fry for another 3 minutes, stirring constantly to ensure nothing can catch and burn.
4. Turn the heat off and stir through the salt and cinnamon, then add the maple syrup mix and stir quickly so it coats the oats, nuts and seeds. Keep stirring as the syrup evaporates and coats everything.
5. Transfer to a bowl and allow to cool. Once it is fully cooled, transfer it to an airtight jar or container and store it for up to 3 weeks.

NOTE You can customize this with your favourite nuts and seeds, or with what you have available. Chopped up walnuts, pistachios, hazelnuts, pecans and cashews all taste great, and you could add hemp seeds, flax seeds, poppy seeds... it's a great way to use up those half-finished packets. If you like dried fruit in your granola you can also stir that in once you have removed the pan from the heat. Dates, cranberries, apricots, coconut flakes and raisins all work well.

PER SERVING: Calories 127 | Fat 5.7g | Sat Fat 0.7g | Carbs 13g | Sugars 4.2g | Fibre 2.9g | Protein 3.9g | Salt 0.25g

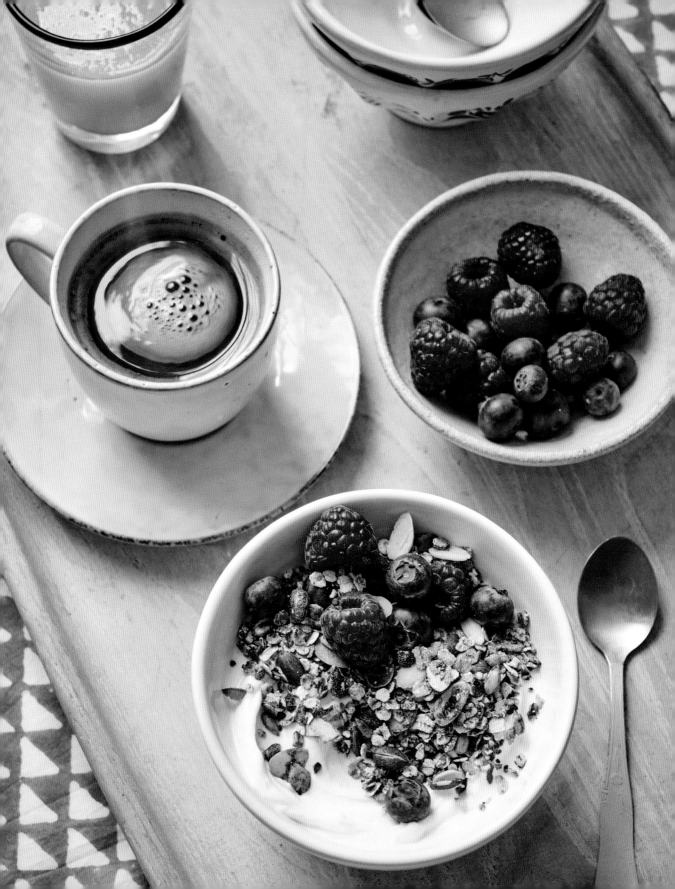

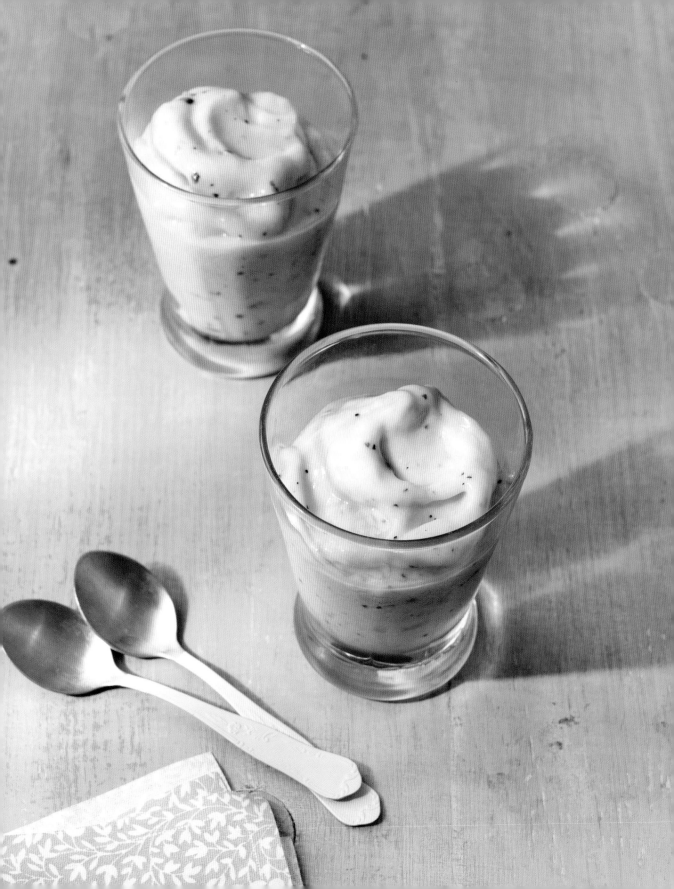

TROPICAL BREAKFAST ICE CREAM

I first made this to try and tempt my daughter into eating breakfast when she started secondary school: she was so nervous in the mornings that she didn't want to eat. It went down a treat and has now become a regular in our household. Frozen mango blends perfectly with cold milk to form a soft-serve ice-cream-type consistency, while passion fruit adds a delicious extra layer of flavour. Using pre-prepared fruit really makes this super-quick and convenient. You will need to use a mini chopper or small food processor for this, as a stick blender usually isn't quite up to the job.

PREP TIME: 2 MINUTES
COOK TIME: NONE

150g (5½oz) frozen mango
  chunks
125ml (4fl oz) chilled semi-
  skimmed milk
1 passion fruit, halved, inside
  scooped out

1. Put the mango chunks, cold milk and passion fruit pulp into a mini chopper and purée until you have a smooth consistency, similar to soft-serve ice cream.
2. Serve immediately. You can freeze any leftovers for another time, but leave it to defrost slightly before eating, so it's soft enough to get a spoon in!

FOR A FROZEN ALTERNATIVE
I always keep bags of frozen mango, raspberries and blueberries in my freezer, as they are so useful for desserts and baking. You can use any frozen fruit that you fancy in this, but be aware that mango is particularly sweet so doesn't need any additional sugar. If I make this with less sweet fruit, I taste it after blending and blend in 1 teaspoon honey if it needs a little extra sweet lift.

PER SERVING: Calories 169 | Fat 2.9g | Sat Fat 1.5g | Carbs 27g | Sugars 26g | Fibre 4.2g | Protein 6g | Salt 0.17g

HONEY ALMOND PORRIDGE
WITH CHIA SEEDS

I absolutely adore the salty-sweet crunch of honey almonds on top of this porridge, which is creamy, dense and satisfying. Chia seeds just add a little extra crunch and texture to regular porridge, and this little breakfast is very filling as well as delicious.

PREP TIME: 2 MINUTES
COOK TIME: 5 MINUTES

60g (2¼oz) jumbo oats
200ml (7fl oz) unsweetened
　almond milk
1 tablespoon chia seeds
1 tablespoon flaked almonds
1 teaspoon honey
salt

1. Put the oats, almond milk and chia seeds in a small saucepan with a little pinch of salt, bring to a simmer and simmer for 5 minutes, stirring occasionally, until the porridge has thickened.
2. Meanwhile, put the flaked almonds in a small frying pan and dry-fry them for 2–3 minutes, stirring regularly, until they look lightly toasted and golden. Add the honey and a pinch of salt to the hot pan, then stir together until the almonds are coated in the honey.
3. Serve the porridge topped with the honey-toasted almonds.

NOTE If you want to add extras to this, fresh raspberries or blueberries or a sliced banana all make great toppings.

PER SERVING: Calories 199 | Fat 7.9g | Sat Fat 0.9g | Carbs 23g | Sugars 3.1g | Fibre 4.6g | Protein 6.8g | Salt 0.62g

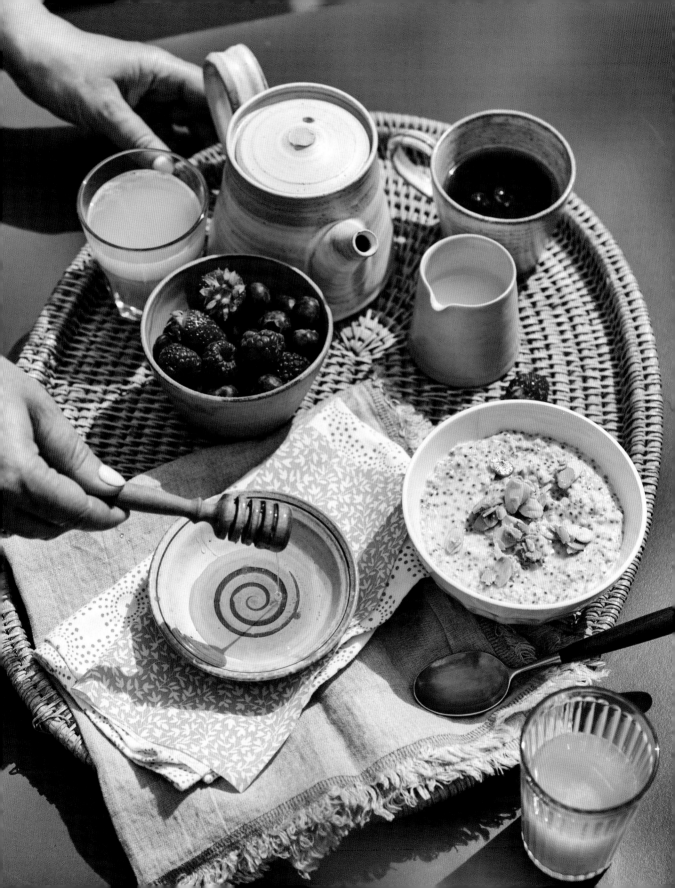

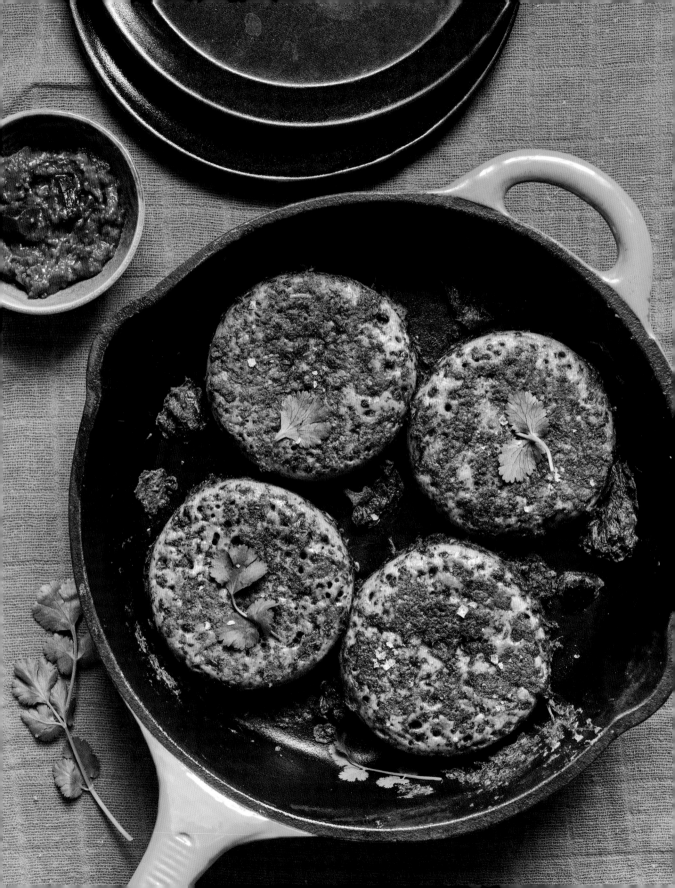

GREEN SPICED CRUMPETS

Bring some Indian-style vibes to brunch with these quick and tasty crumpets. They are the perfect vehicle for eggs, and some simple flavours and bright green colour whizzed into the eggs here takes the idea to the next level. Serve these with your condiment of choice: mango chutney, aubergine pickle, chilli sauce and brown sauce all work well.

PREP TIME: 5 MINUTES
COOK TIME: 4–5 MINUTES

2 eggs
1 green chilli, halved and deseeded
small handful of baby spinach leaves
small handful of coriander, plus extra leaves to serve
½ teaspoon ground cumin
½ teaspoon ground turmeric
spray oil
4 crumpets
salt and pepper, to taste

1. Put the eggs, chilli, spinach, coriander, cumin, turmeric and salt and pepper into a mini chopper and whizz up until everything is very finely chopped, almost puréed.
2. Pour the egg mixture into a large shallow dish, such as an oven dish or roasting pan. One at a time, place the crumpets (holey side down) into the mixture and press down with a fork until they are saturated with egg.
3. Spray a large non-stick frying pan with oil, place over a medium heat and allow to heat for 10–20 seconds before placing the eggy crumpets into the pan. Pour any remaining egg mixture over the top of the crumpets, and once they start sizzling, increase the heat and cook for 2 minutes on each side until the egg has cooked through. You know they are ready when you push down on them with a spatula and no liquid comes out.
4. Serve with your condiment of choice (see introduction) and scattered with coriander leaves.

NOTE Aubergine pickle is delicious with this and is becoming more readily available in supermarkets in the UK. It has a rich, spicy, earthy, sweet and salty taste. It's also great in cheese sandwiches in place of your regular sandwich pickle.

PER SERVING: Calories 281 | Fat 6.5g | Sat Fat 1.7g | Carbs 40g | Sugars 2.4g | Fibre 2.5g | Protein 14g | Salt 2.1g

PESTO FRIED EGGS WITH MUSHROOMS ON MUFFINS

Pesto fried eggs are a great way to make a brunch taste and look great – try them with my homemade Pestos (see pages 128–133). I have served them here over a toasted wholemeal English muffin, which is one of my favourite weekend breakfast treats, but you can serve them however you like!

PREP TIME: 2 MINUTES
COOK TIME: 7 MINUTES

½ teaspoon unsalted butter
100g (3½oz) chestnut
   mushrooms, sliced
spray oil
2 teaspoons pesto
2 eggs
1 wholemeal English muffin,
   sliced in half
salt and pepper, to taste
finely chopped parsley leaves,
   to serve

1. Melt the butter in a nonstick frying pan (for which you have a lid) and fry the mushrooms for 4 minutes. Season them with salt and pepper and set them aside in a small bowl.
2. Lightly spray the frying pan with oil, then add 2 teaspoons of pesto either side of the pan and use the back of the spoon to spread them into circles. Increase the heat to medium and cook until the pesto starts to sizzle (30–60 seconds), then crack an egg on top of each circle of pesto.
3. Put a lid on the frying pan. Toast the muffin while you wait for the eggs to cook to your liking (see below). Place the toasted muffin on a plate.
4. Spoon the mushrooms and any juices from their bowl over the toasted muffin halves, then use a spatula to remove the eggs from the frying pan and place on top of the mushrooms. Season with salt and pepper, sprinkle with parsley and serve.

FOR PERFECT FRIED EGGS
To avoid using too much butter or oil, you really need a nonstick pan. For a sunny-side-up egg with a runny yolk, cook for about 3 minutes with a lid on (the steam will cook the white). For an over-easy egg (or if you don't have a lid), after 3 minutes flip it over and cook for 1 more minute.

PER SERVING: Calories 443 | Fat 26g | Sat Fat 8.9g | Carbs 27g | Sugars 11g | Fibre 6.1g | Protein 21g | Salt 2.2g

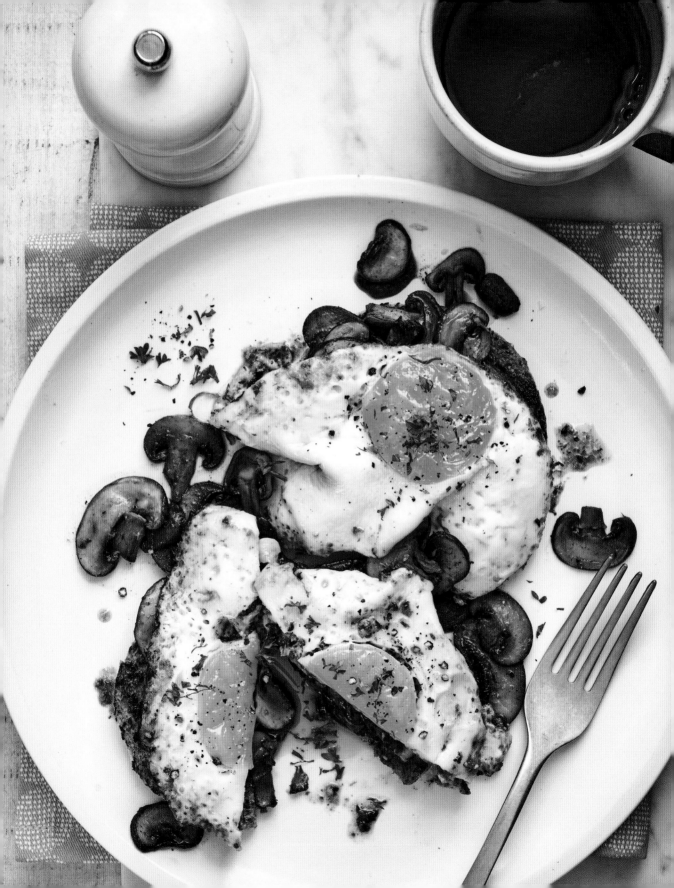

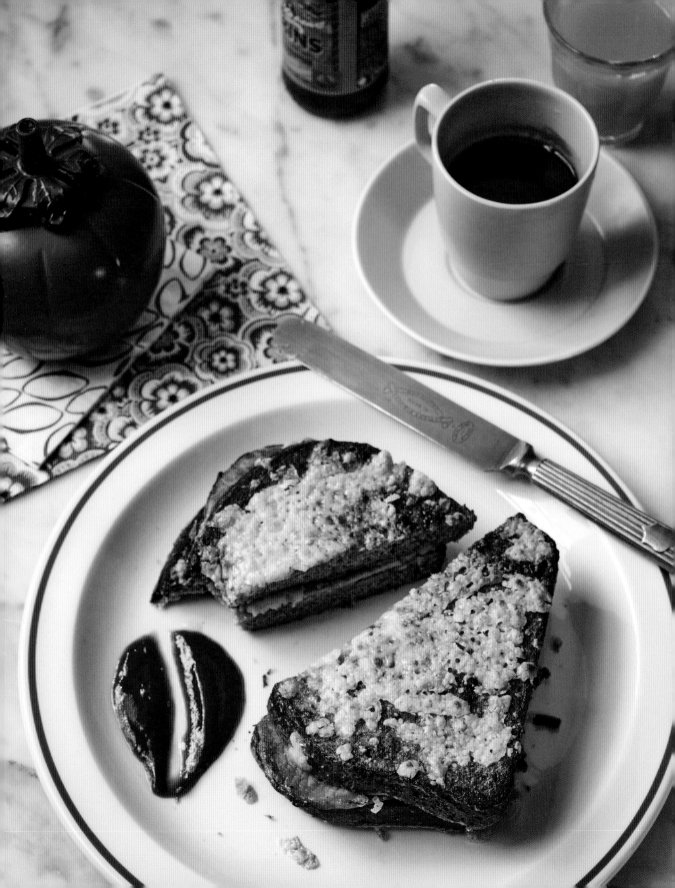

CHEESE & BACON EGGY BREAD TOASTIES

We love sweet eggy bread in our household, but this savoury toastie hits the spot perfectly when you fancy a good, filling, indulgent-tasting brunch.

PREP TIME: 3 MINUTES
COOK TIME: 8 MINUTES

4 bacon medallions
spray oil
2 eggs, lightly beaten
4 slices of wholemeal bread
60g (2¼oz) Cheddar cheese, grated
a few dashes of Worcestershire sauce
pepper, to taste

1. Place the bacon medallions under a hot grill for 5 minutes.
2. Meanwhile, spray a large nonstick frying pan with oil (if it isn't big enough to hold all 4 slices of bread, you may need to use 2 pans) and place over a medium-high heat. Put the eggs in a shallow bowl, season them with pepper and soak each slice of bread in the egg on both sides.
3. Once all the bread is coated in egg, fry the first side for about 2 minutes, then flip each piece over with a spatula, and sprinkle half the grated Cheddar over 2 of the slices. Fry for about 2 more minutes until the egg is cooked through (this will depend on how thick the bread is).
4. Remove the grill pan from the oven and remove the bacon. Put the 2 cheese-covered slices of eggy bread on the grill pan. Place 2 pieces of cooked bacon on each cheesy slice, then lay the other piece of eggy bread on top. Now sprinkle the remaining Cheddar over the top of each sandwich, add the Worcestershire sauce and pop back under the grill.
5. Grill for about 3 minutes until the cheese on top is golden brown and bubbling. Cut each sandwich in half and serve.

FOR A VEGETARIAN ALTERNATIVE
Fry a sliced field mushroom in a separate pan while the eggy bread is cooking and add to the sandwich instead of the bacon. Replace the Worcestershire sauce (which usually contains anchovies) with a splash of balsamic vinegar or soy sauce.

PER SERVING: Calories 485 | Fat 21g | Sat Fat 9g | Carbs 32g | Sugars 2.9g | Fibre 5.6g | Protein 38g | Salt 4g

LITTLE HAM, LEEK & CHEDDAR FRITTATAS

Perfect picnic food, or a grab-and-go breakfast or healthy snack, these mini frittatas are great to have on hand.

PREP TIME: 5 MINUTES

COOK TIME: 14 MINUTES

4 eggs

60g (2¼oz) Cheddar cheese, grated

2 slices of ham, finely chopped

1 leek, trimmed, outer leaves discarded, finely chopped (see note on page 43)

low-calorie cooking spray (optional)

1 teaspoon dried oregano

salt and pepper, to taste

1. Preheat the oven to 210°C/190°C fan (410°F), Gas Mark 6½.
2. In a bowl, lightly beat the eggs and add the Cheddar, ham, leek and some salt and pepper.
3. Place 6 muffin cases into a muffin tray and spray them with low-calorie cooking spray, or use silicone muffin cases. Divide the egg mixture between the cases, making sure the goodies within are evenly shared.
4. Sprinkle the top of each with a little oregano, then pop into the oven and bake for 14 minutes.
5. Allow to cool slightly before removing from the cases. These are delicious warm or cold.

NOTE You can mix these up with some of your favourite flavour combinations, or keep them meat-free if you prefer. You can replace the Cheddar with grated mozzarella, or finely chopped feta, or use some different dried herbs, such as thyme. Use spring onions instead of leeks, or add peas, finely chopped red peppers or sliced asparagus spears. These are also a great way to use up any small amounts of vegetables or fresh herbs left in the refrigerator.

PER FRITTATA: Calories 107 | Fat 7.4g | Sat Fat 3.3g | Carbs 1g | Sugars 0.5g | Fibre 0.5g | Protein 8.9g | Salt 0.6g

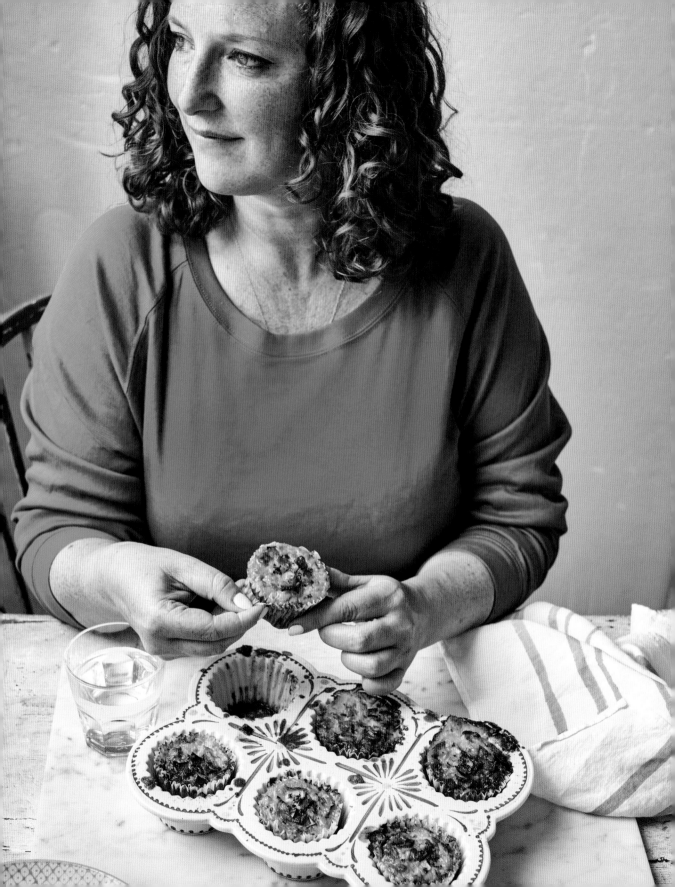

CHAPTER 2

MEAT-FREE DAYS

GOLDEN GRILLED CHEESY LEEKS

This is a hearty vegetarian main course that takes no time at all to prepare. I happily eat a bowl of this on its own, or you can serve it with some green vegetables such as broccoli, green beans or asparagus, or fresh bread. It also makes a tasty side dish for meat or fish.

PREP TIME: 5 MINUTES
COOK TIME: 20 MINUTES

1 teaspoon unsalted butter
2 leeks, trimmed, cleaned and
   sliced (see note on page 43)
2 garlic cloves, crushed
2 × 400g (14oz) cans of cannellini
   beans, drained and rinsed
100ml (3½fl oz) semi-skimmed
   milk
100ml (3½fl oz) hot vegetable
   stock
1 small cauliflower, cut into
   bite-sized pieces
1 teaspoon salt
½ teaspoon dried thyme, plus
   extra to serve (optional)
½ teaspoon dried rosemary,
   plus extra to serve (optional)
½ teaspoon pepper
60g (2¼oz) mature Cheddar
   cheese, grated
10g (¼oz) Parmesan-style
   vegetarian cheese, finely grated
finely chopped parsley leaves,
   to serve (optional)

1. Melt the butter in a sauté pan (for which you have a lid), add the leeks and garlic and fry over a medium-high heat for 5 minutes, stirring occasionally.
2. Add the cannellini beans, milk, hot stock, cauliflower, salt, thyme, rosemary and pepper and stir it all together. Pop the lid on and simmer for 10 minutes.
3. Preheat the grill to high, remove the lid of the pan and stir through the Cheddar. (If your pan is not flameproof, then transfer everything to a flameproof baking dish at this point.) Scatter the Parmesan-style cheese over the top and grill for 5 minutes to melt the cheese and slightly char the top layer.
4. Serve immediately, scattered with chopped parsley or more dried herbs, if you like.

NOTE If you want to add a meat element to this, then fry some finely sliced chorizo or smoked bacon with the leeks for the first 5 minutes.

PER SERVING: Calories 253 | Fat 9.5g | Sat Fat 5.5g | Carbs 24g | Sugars 6.8g | Fibre 7.5g | Protein 1.5g | Salt 2.7g

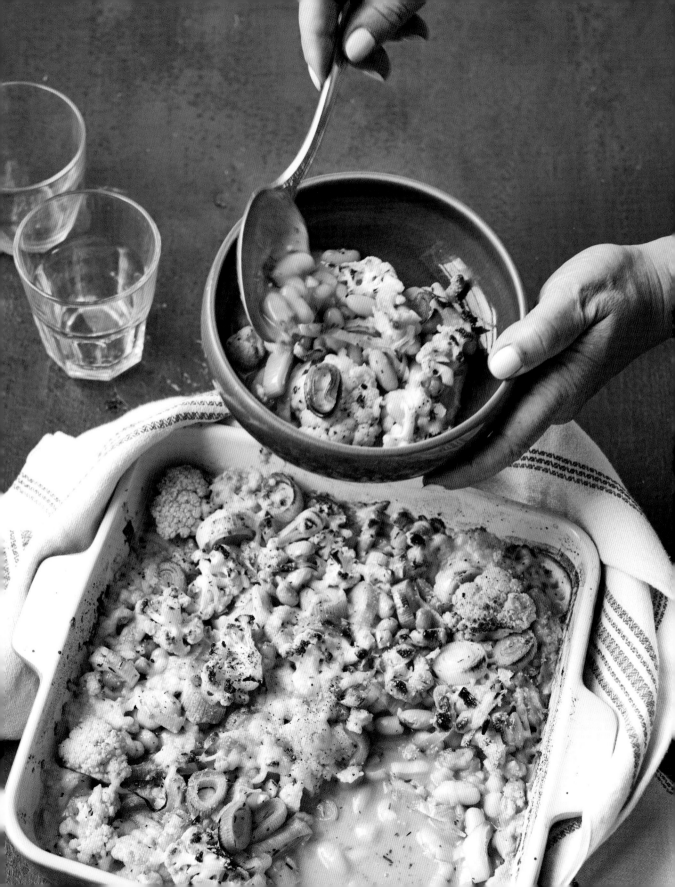

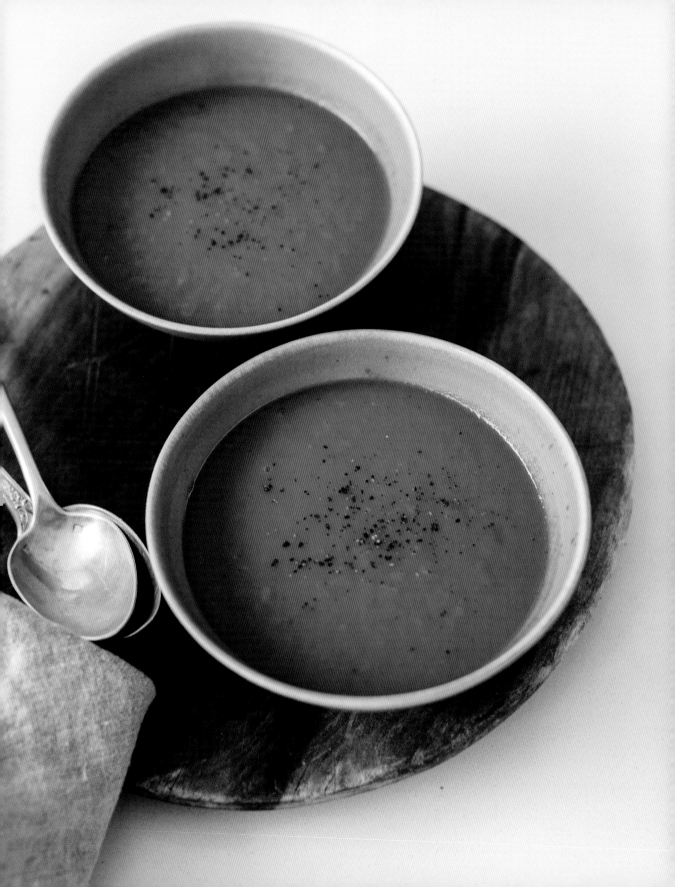

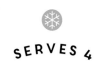

BLOODY MARY SOUP

This is the soup you need when you are feeling a bit under the weather: it's a lovely, warming pick-me-up. I have to admit I don't actually like Bloody Mary cocktails, but I could eat this every day. Add the vodka if you fancy, leave it out if you don't; both ways are delicious.

PREP TIME: 2 MINUTES
COOK TIME: 15 MINUTES

spray oil
2 celery sticks, finely chopped
2 × 400g (14oz) cans of chopped tomatoes
600ml (20fl oz) hot vegetable stock
2 tablespoons Worcestershire sauce
1 tablespoon tomato purée
1 teaspoon sugar
½ teaspoon celery salt
a few dashes of Tabasco sauce, to taste
2 tablespoons vodka (optional)
1 lemon wedge
salt and pepper, to taste

1. Spray a saucepan with oil and fry the celery for 5 minutes over a medium heat, stirring occasionally.
2. Add the chopped tomatoes, hot stock, Worcestershire sauce, tomato purée, sugar, celery salt and Tabasco and allow to simmer vigorously for 10 minutes.
3. Stir in the vodka, if using, a couple of minutes before you remove the pan from the heat.
4. Squeeze in the juice from the lemon wedge, then use a stick blender to blend it all into a smooth soup. Adjust the seasoning to taste and serve.

MAKE YOUR OWN CELERY SALT
Celery salt is usually easy to source, but it's easy to make your own. Simply remove the leaves from a head of celery, then lay them out on a baking tray. Bake at 200°C/180°C fan (400°F), Gas Mark 6 for 5–10 minutes, or until dried out but not burned or scorched. When they are cool, use your fingers to crumble them, discarding any parts that aren't crispy. Mix them together with an equal quantity of fine sea salt or sea salt flakes, and store in an airtight jar.

PER SERVING: Calories 114 | Fat 1.4g | Sat Fat 0.1g | Carbs 17g | Sugars 16g | Fibre 3.8g | Protein 4.5g | Salt 2.2g

TASTE THE RAINBOW NOODLE SALAD

A no-cook, fruity and peanutty dressing for noodles and crunchy vegetables that is light, fresh and quick to make. This makes a great summer salad, barbecue dish or an easy lunch for work.

PREP TIME: 10 MINUTES
COOK TIME: 4 MINUTES

1 orange, zest and pith cut away,
   roughly chopped (see note)
1 lime, zest and pith cut away,
   roughly chopped (see note)
1 garlic clove
1 tablespoon smooth peanut
   butter
1 tablespoon soy sauce
1 tablespoon honey
200g (7oz) fine or medium egg
   noodles
¼ red cabbage, shredded
2 carrots, grated
3 spring onions, sliced
1 red chilli, deseeded and finely
   chopped
small handful of coriander,
   finely chopped

1. Put the orange and the lime in a mini chopper or small food processor with the garlic, peanut butter, soy sauce and honey. Blend until smooth.

2. Cook the noodles according to the packet instructions (usually around 4 minutes), then drain and rinse them through with cold water.

3. In a large bowl, toss together the noodles, cabbage and carrots, pour in the dressing and toss everything together again until the vegetables and noodles are coated in the dressing.

4. Serve scattered with the spring onions, red chilli and coriander.

NOTE To prepare the orange and lime, place the fruit on a chopping board, and, using a sharp knife, slice about 1cm (½ inch) off the top and bottom. Stand it up so that the flesh is exposed at the top, then begin to cut the skin off, following the curved contour of the fruit and cutting just underneath the white pith to remove it all. Repeat this all around the fruit until there is no zest or pith remaining.

PER SERVING: Calories 272 | Fat 3.8g | Sat Fat 0.8g | Carbs 47g | Sugars 14g | Fibre 5.7g | Protein 9.2g | Salt 1.3g

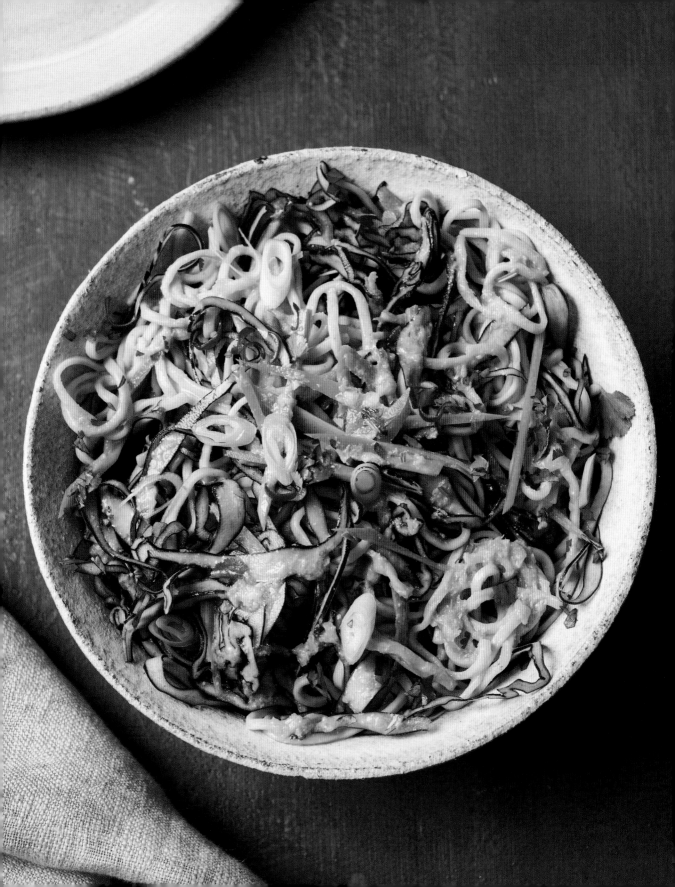

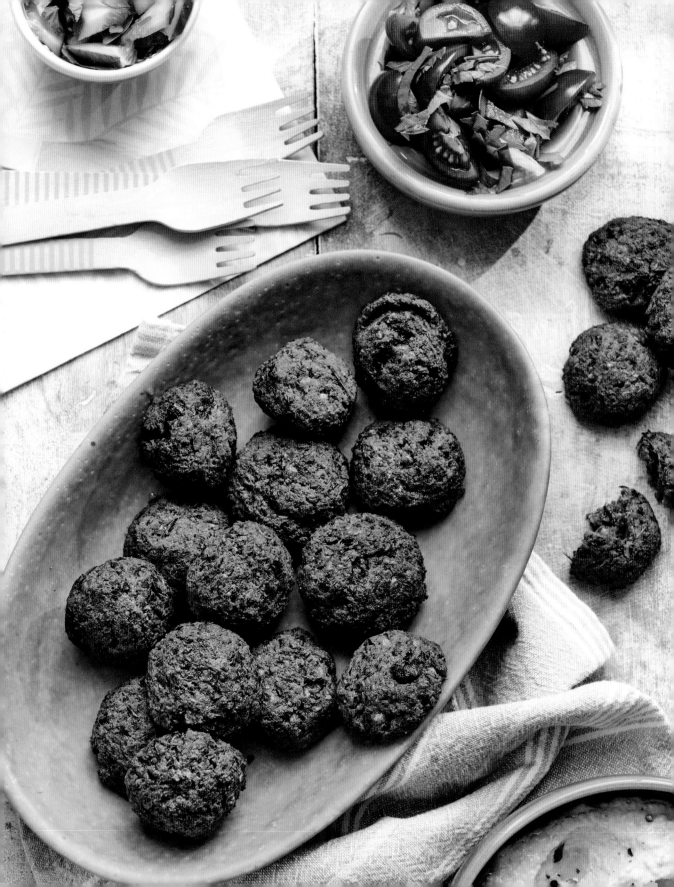

BEETROOT, KALE & CHILLI FALAFEL

Flavoursome falafel with earthy, sharp beetroot and a chilli kick, these make great snacks and light lunches. Serve with salads, couscous, in pittas or with a hummus dip.

PREP TIME: 10 MINUTES
COOK TIME: 15–20 MINUTES

400g (14oz) can of chickpeas, drained and rinsed
100g (3½oz) steamed beetroot
3 garlic cloves
½ small red onion
2 large handfuls of kale leaves, coarse stalks removed
small handful of parsley leaves and stalks
juice of ½ lemon
2 teaspoons ground cumin
1 teaspoon ground coriander
½ teaspoon salt
½ teaspoon chilli flakes
2 tablespoons plain flour
1 tablespoon olive oil

1. Preheat the oven to 240°C/220°C fan (475°F), Gas Mark 9. Line a large baking tray with nonstick baking paper.
2. Put all the ingredients in a food processor bowl, then blend until you have a smooth mixture.
3. Shape the mixture into balls, about 3cm (1¼ inches) in diameter; you should get about 20 falafel. Place them on the prepared baking tray as they are formed.
4. Bake in the oven for 15–20 minutes: check on them after 15 minutes and if they look like they need a bit more crisping up (and are not starting to burn), then give them a few more minutes.
5. Allow to cool and harden up slightly before serving. Serve warm or cold.

NOTE This is a great recipe for using up leftover kale, as it can sometimes be a challenge to get through a whole bag of it!

PER SERVING: Calories 168 | Fat 5.3g | Sat Fat 0.7g | Carbs 21g | Sugars 3.8g | Fibre 4.5g | Protein 6.7g | Salt 0.7g

PEA, SPINACH, MINT & GREEN CHILLI SOUP

This soup is just so quick and easy to make, you really can't beat it for a quick option. Neither frozen peas nor spinach need much cooking at all, and cool mint with spicy chilli makes a great combination for a really enjoyable but healthy soup. If you are feeling extra-hungry, then this really is delicious served alongside wholemeal toast with bubbling cheese grilled on top.

PREP TIME: 5 MINUTES
COOK TIME: 10 MINUTES

spray oil
1 small onion, finely chopped
2 garlic cloves, crushed
1 green chilli, deseeded and
    chopped
500ml (18fl oz) hot vegetable
    stock
400g (14oz) frozen garden peas
2 large handfuls of baby spinach
    leaves
small handful of mint leaves,
    plus extra small leaves to serve
salt and pepper, to taste

TO SERVE (OPTIONAL)
swirl of fat-free Greek yogurt
a sprinkle of nigella seeds

1. Spray a saucepan (for which you have a lid) with oil and sweat the onion, garlic and chilli over a medium-low heat for 5 minutes with the lid on, stirring occasionally.
2. Pour in the hot stock, add the peas and bring to the boil. Reduce the heat to a simmer, stir in the spinach and allow to simmer for 5 minutes.
3. Remove from the heat, add the mint leaves, and, using a stick blender, blend the soup until it is a smooth consistency. Season to taste with salt and pepper.
4. Add a swirl of fat-free Greek yogurt, a few small mint leaves and a little sprinkle of black pepper or nigella seeds to serve, if you like.

NOTE Frozen vegetables are an absolutely brilliant thing to keep in the freezer for quick soups such as this. You can even buy pre-chopped frozen onion, which works perfectly in soups, stews and curries. Make the most of these types of healthy convenience foods to save on time, while still cooking from scratch.

PER SERVING: Calories 207 | Fat 2.1g | Sat Fat 0.4g | Carbs 28g | Sugars 16g | Fibre 13g | Protein 13g | Salt 1.9g

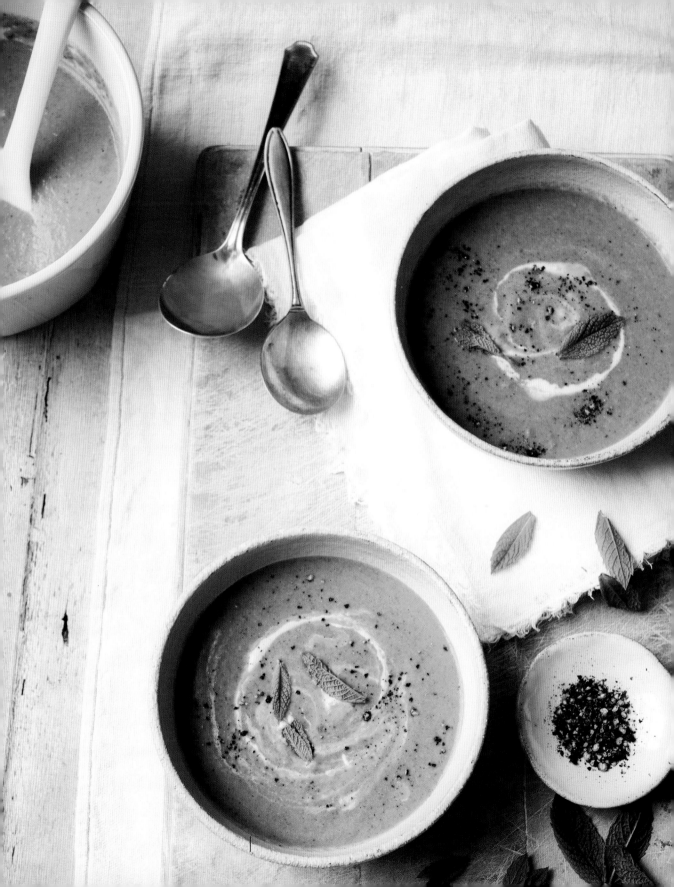

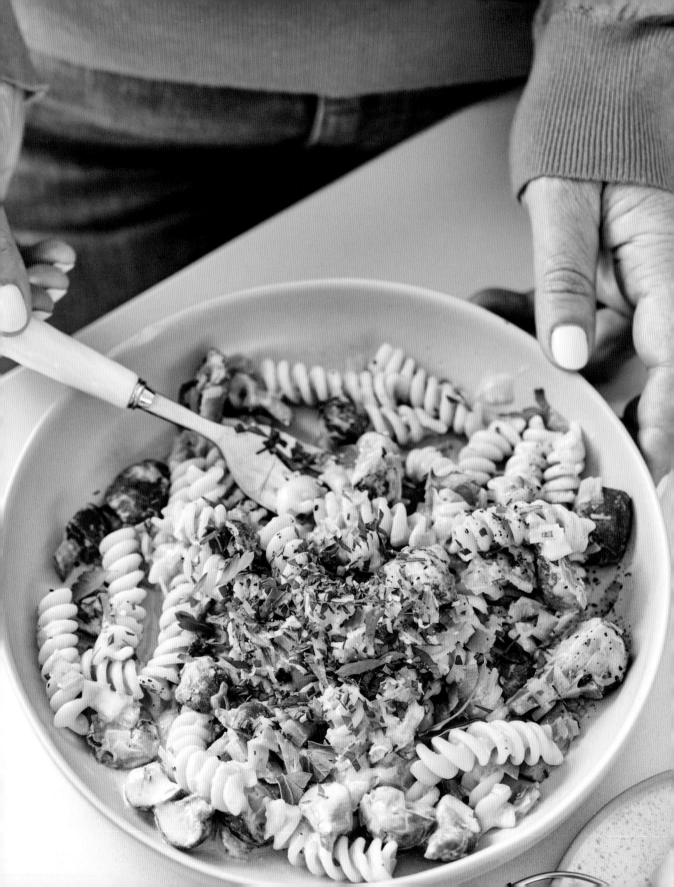

LEEK, MUSHROOM & ROSEMARY FUSILLI

A super-speedy, light and simple sauce with sweet leeks, earthy mushrooms and a hint of rosemary and lemon. Cutting the chestnut mushrooms into quarters gives great texture to this meat-free dish. Serve with extra steamed green vegetables on the side.

PREP TIME: 5 MINUTES
COOK TIME: 12 MINUTES

300g (10½oz) fusilli pasta
spray oil
3 leeks, trimmed, cleaned and
    sliced (see note)
300g (10½oz) chestnut
    mushrooms, quartered
2 garlic cloves, crushed
leaves from 2 rosemary sprigs,
    finely chopped
1 teaspoon coarse salt
juice of 1 lemon
2 tablespoons half-fat crème
    fraîche
10g (¼oz) Parmesan-style
    vegetarian cheese, finely grated
coarsely ground black pepper,
    to taste
handful of parsley leaves, finely
    chopped, to serve

1. Cook the pasta in a large pan of boiling water and set a timer for 11 minutes.
2. Spray a sauté pan with oil and add the leeks, mushrooms, garlic, rosemary and coarse salt. Fry gently while the pasta cooks, stirring occasionally.
3. When the pasta has 2 minutes left to cook, add the lemon juice to the leeks and mushrooms and stir through.
4. When the timer goes off, drain the pasta, reserving a little of the cooking water
5. Tip the cooked pasta and reserved water into the pan with the leek and mushroom mixture, spoon in the crème fraîche and cheese, then mix everything together to coat the pasta in the light sauce.
6. Serve with coarsely ground black pepper and parsley scattered on top.

NOTE Leeks often trap dirt between their layers. To ensure a nice clean leek, first trim off the roots and the tougher green leaves at the top, plus the outer layer if it feels tough (you can save these for making stock or soup). Next, halve the leek lengthways, then hold it under running water to rinse away any soil or grit. For this dish, I cut each half of the leek into half again, lengthways, then finely slice it ready for frying.

PER SERVING: Calories 330 | Fat 5.8g | Sat Fat 2.7g | Carbs 55g | Sugars 4.8g | Fibre 5.7g | Protein 12g | Salt 1.3g

MOZZARELLA & SUNDRIED TOMATO RISOTTO

A family favourite, this risotto has a creamy texture, with oozing melted mozzarella and pops of flavour from sundried tomatoes and basil. Risotto needs your attention while it's cooking (see tips, below), but this recipe needs very little prep. It is lovely served with rocket or asparagus (or both).

PREP TIME: 5 MINUTES
COOK TIME: 25 MINUTES

1.5 litres (2½ pints) hot vegetable stock
spray oil
1 onion, finely chopped
50g (1¾oz) sundried tomatoes, drained and patted with kitchen paper to remove oil, then finely sliced
300g (10½oz) carnaroli or arborio risotto rice
175g (6oz) mozzarella cheese, chopped into small cubes
handful of basil leaves, finely shredded, plus extra to serve
pepper, to taste
15g Parmesan-style vegetarian cheese, finely grated, to serve

1. Pour the vegetable stock into a saucepan and set over a very low heat to keep it hot.
2. Spray a deep sauté pan with oil and stir-fry the onion over a medium heat for 5 minutes.
3. Stir the tomatoes and risotto rice into the onion pan, then add a ladleful of stock and stir. Once it's absorbed add another ladleful.
4. Add the remaining stock, a ladleful at a time, and cook until the rice is al dente, stirring regularly (see tips, below) for 15–20 minutes.
5. Try the rice to check that it is al dente; it should be a little bit chewy, but not gritty. Stir through the mozzarella and basil and season with pepper, then scatter with the grated cheese and basil leaves and serve immediately.

TIPS FOR SUCCESSFUL RISOTTO
- Don't wash the rice first, as its starch helps to make the risotto creamy.
- Stir the rice often, but not constantly. Stirring helps release the starch from the rice and prevents it sticking to the base of the pan, but too much stirring can cool it down and lengthen the cooking time.
- Don't add all the stock at once, this will just boil the rice and won't create that creamy risotto consistency.

PER SERVING: Calories 485 | Fat 14g | Sat Fat 7.3g | Carbs 70g | Sugars 8.7g | Fibre 4.7g | Protein 17g | Salt 3.2g

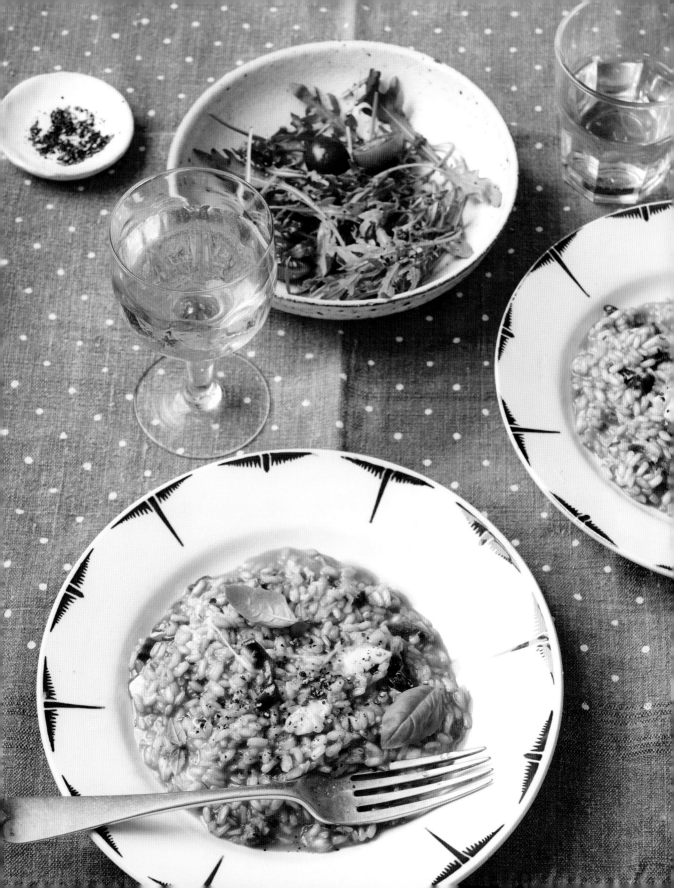

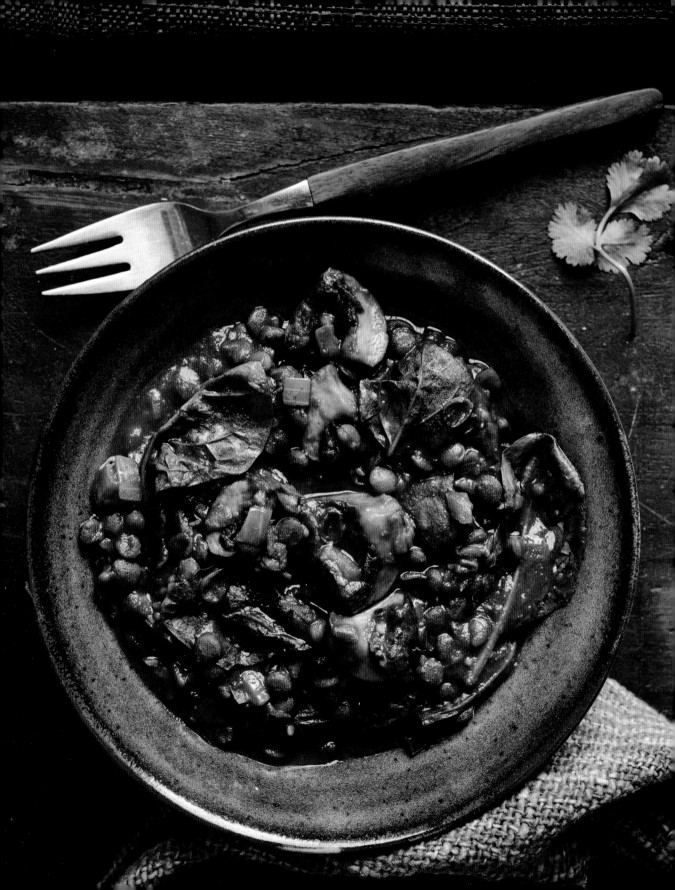

FIERY GARLIC MUSHROOM & LENTIL DAL

Filling, satisfying and nutritious, this is the best sort of bowl food and is ideal to reheat for quick lunches. You can serve it with rice if you wish, but it's lovely as a stand-alone dish.

PREP TIME: 5 MINUTES
COOK TIME: 15 MINUTES

FOR THE SPICE MIX
1 teaspoon garam masala
1 teaspoon ground turmeric
1 teaspoon mustard seeds
1 teaspoon cumin seeds
1 teaspoon salt
½ teaspoon chilli powder

FOR THE DAL
1 teaspoon unsalted butter
1 onion, finely chopped
300g (10½oz) chestnut
   mushrooms, quartered
2 bird's eye chillies, deseeded
   and finely chopped
4 garlic cloves, crushed
500ml (18fl oz) hot vegetable
   stock
2 tablespoons tomato purée
2 × 400g (14oz) cans of green
   lentils, drained and rinsed
3 large handfuls of baby spinach
   leaves
coriander leaves, to serve
   (optional)

1. Make up the spice mix by mixing all the ingredients in a small bowl, so that it is ready to go.
2. Melt the butter in a sauté pan, add the onion and fry for 3 minutes, stirring occasionally.
3. Add the mushrooms, bird's eye chillies and garlic to the pan, stir for about 30 seconds, then add the spice mix and stir-fry for 1 minute.
4. Pour in the hot stock, add the tomato purée and lentils, stir, then simmer for 10 minutes.
5. Add the spinach and stir through until wilted.
6. Serve scattered with coriander leaves if you like.

A TIP FOR EXTRA FLAVOUR
If you ever make a curry that tastes a little bitter, just stir through 1–2 teaspoons mango chutney which will instantly counteract the bitterness and give it a lovely little extra layer of flavour. (But remember it will also increase the calories.)

PER SERVING: Calories 192 | Fat 3.4g | Sat Fat 1.7g | Carbs 22g | Sugars 6g | Fibre 14g | Protein 11g | Salt 2.2g

SPICY BLACK BEAN BURGERS

I was very sceptical that a meat-free burger could be as satisfying as a beef one, but these really hit the spot. They have great flavour and a satisfying consistency. Using a food processor means that they only take minutes to make, while oven-baking allows you to prepare any other fillings or side dishes while they cook.

PREP TIME: 8 MINUTES
COOK TIME: 20 MINUTES

80g (2¾oz) porridge oats

1 carrot, roughly chopped

1 red chilli, deseeded, or keep the
    seeds in for extra spice

large handful of coriander leaves

2 spring onions, roughly chopped

1 teaspoon garlic granules

½ teaspoon ground cumin

½ teaspoon smoked paprika

½ teaspoon salt

400g (14oz) can of black beans,
    drained and rinsed

1 tablespoon soy sauce

1 tablespoon tomato ketchup

spray oil

TO SERVE

4 wholemeal buns

burger toppings of choice
    (see note)

1. Preheat the oven to 220°C/200°C fan (425°F), Gas Mark 7. Line a baking tray with nonstick baking paper.

2. Place the oats in a food processor bowl and whizz them to break them down.

3. Add the carrot, chilli, coriander, spring onions, garlic granules, cumin, smoked paprika and salt and blend again until there are no large chunks.

4. Add the black beans, soy sauce and ketchup, then pulse-blend to partially break down the beans (don't pureé them too finely, as you want some texture).

5. Shape the mixture into 4 burger patties with your hands, then lay them on the prepared tray and spray lightly with oil. If you want to freeze these, it's best to do it – with nonstick baking paper separating each patty – before cooking or spraying with oil.

6. Bake for 20 minutes, checking on them after 15 minutes just to make sure they aren't burning.

7. Serve in wholemeal buns with toppings of your choice.

NOTE Some ideas for burger toppings: cheese, salsa (try my Dark & Smoky Chipotle Salsa, see page 162), lettuce, tomato, cucumber, fried egg, onions, ketchup, coleslaw… or try something really different and spread a little bit of peanut butter inside the bun: delicious!

PER SERVING: Calories 254 | Fat 2.3g | Sat Fat 0.4g | Carbs 41g | Sugars 8.7g | Fibre 10g | Protein 11g | Salt 2.2g

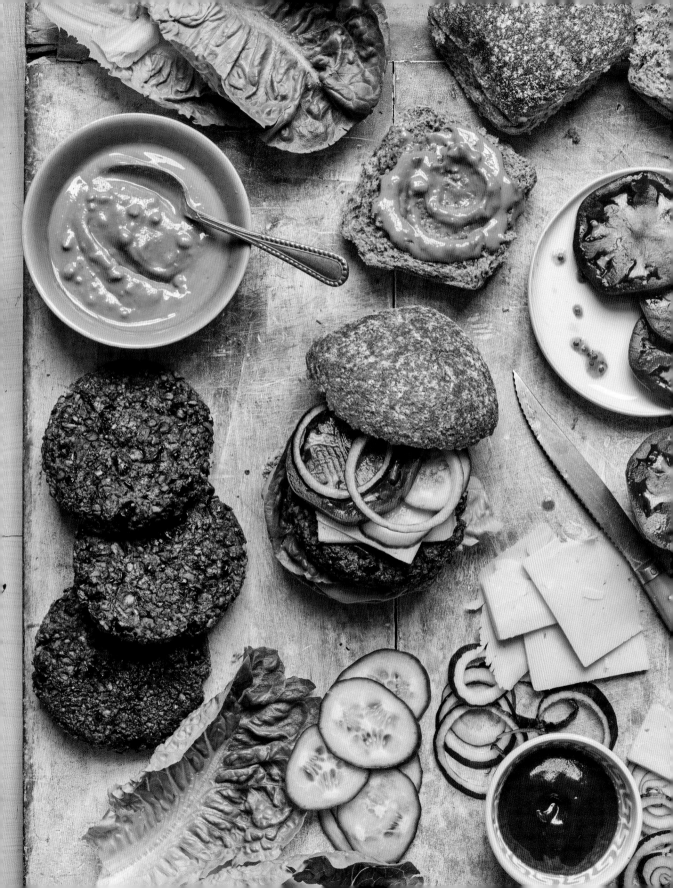

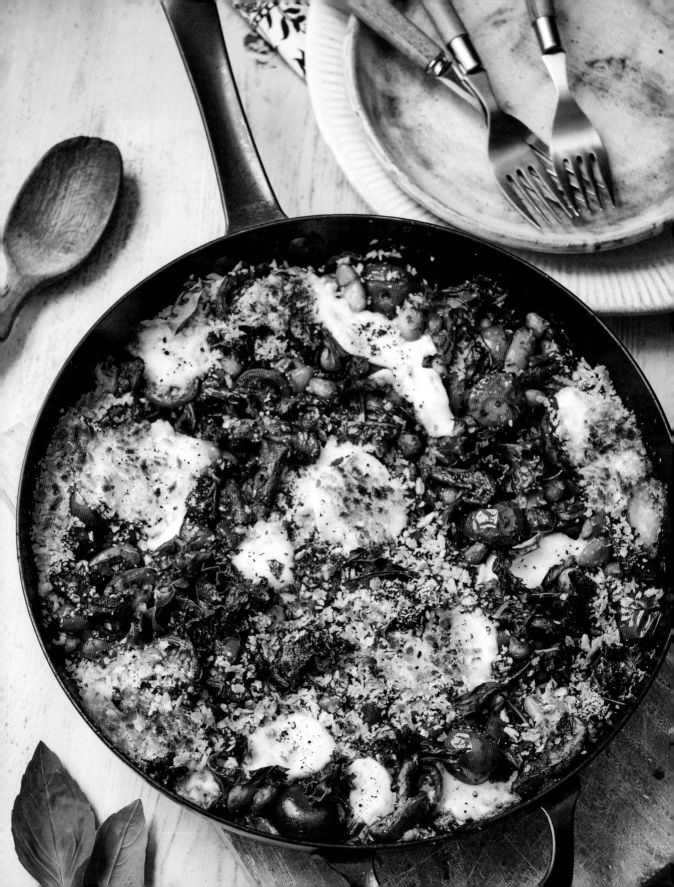

ITALIAN-STYLE BORLOTTI BEAN GRATIN

**A truly hearty meal, this uses some of my favourite Italian flavours.
Melted mozzarella and a breadcrumb crunch really top it off.**

PREP TIME: 10 MINUTES
COOK TIME: 20 MINUTES

spray oil
1 red onion, finely chopped
3 garlic cloves, crushed
1 red pepper, deseeded and finely
  chopped
150g (5½oz) mushrooms, sliced
150g (5½oz) cherry tomatoes,
  halved
large handful of kale leaves,
  coarse stalks removed,
  roughly chopped
400g (14oz) can of borlotti
  beans, drained and rinsed
1 tablespoon smoked paprika
1 tablespoon Italian-style mixed
  dried herbs
½ teaspoon chilli flakes
  (optional)
½ teaspoon fennel seeds
½ teaspoon salt
½ teaspoon pepper
1 tablespoon tomato purée
1 tablespoon balsamic vinegar
handful of basil leaves, torn
125g (4½oz) mozzarella cheese
25g (1oz) panko breadcrumbs

1. Spray a flameproof sauté pan with oil and fry the onion,
   garlic, red pepper and mushrooms for 5 minutes, stirring
   occasionally.
2. Add the tomatoes, kale, borlotti beans, smoked paprika,
   dried herbs, chilli flakes, fennel seeds, salt and pepper,
   tomato purée and balsamic vinegar and simmer for
   10 minutes, stirring every now and again.
3. Preheat the grill to high. Stir the basil into the pan. Tear
   the mozzarella and arrange it on top, then scatter the
   breadcrumbs over. Season with a little salt and pepper.
4. Grill for 5 minutes, to allow the mozzarella to melt and
   the breadcrumbs to toast, then serve. You can freeze any
   leftovers, or, if you're making it for the freezer, spoon the
   mixture into a baking dish and freeze it before scattering
   over the mozzarella and breadcrumbs.

NOTE This is a great dish for using up bits and pieces of
leftover vegetables in the refrigerator, as most things will
work well. You could add spinach, green beans, peas, broccoli,
cauliflower, cooked carrot, extra peppers, shallots, asparagus,
celery, aubergines or courgettes.

PER SERVING: Calories 210 | Fat 7.8g | Sat Fat 4.6g | Carbs 58g | Sugars 20g | Fibre 4.7g | Protein 13g | Salt 1g

SMASHED BROCCOLI CONCHIGLIE

The simplest of pasta sauces. Although in most circumstances I would avoid overcooked broccoli, in this Italian-inspired dish it is cooked until it's able to be fully broken down and then just very lightly flavoured with lemon, chilli and cheese. It then forms a satisfyingly tasty concoction that clings to the pasta shells to make a light and fresh-tasting sauce.

PREP TIME: 5 MINUTES
COOK TIME: 20 MINUTES

spray oil
3 garlic cloves, crushed
1 head of broccoli, broken into
   florets
250ml (9fl oz) vegetable stock
300g (10½oz) conchiglie pasta
   (shells)
1 teaspoon Italian-style mixed
   dried herbs
½ teaspoon chilli flakes
finely grated zest and juice of
   1 lemon
20g (¾oz) Parmesan-style
   vegetarian cheese, finely grated
salt and pepper, to taste

1. Spray a sauté pan (for which you have a lid) with oil and fry the garlic for 30 seconds, then add the broccoli and vegetable stock, place the lid on the pan and bring to the boil, then reduce the heat to a simmer and leave simmering for 15 minutes.

2. Meanwhile, cook the pasta in a large pan of boiling water for about 12 minutes until al dente. Remove the lid from the broccoli pan and give it a stir.

3. Drain the pasta, reserving a little of the cooking water, and set aside while you finish the sauce.

4. Use a wooden spoon or potato masher to break down the broccoli: it should easily mash right down. If you need a little more liquid, add some of the pasta water.

5. Stir the mixed herbs, chilli, lemon zest and juice and cheese into the broccoli. Season with salt and pepper.

6. Stir the pasta through the sauce until it's thoroughly coated, then serve in warmed pasta bowls.

NOTE Fancy a bit of crunch with this? Toast some sunflower seeds and pumpkin seeds in a dry frying pan for a few minutes, then scatter them over the top of the pasta.

PER SERVING: Calories 322 | Fat 3.7g | Sat Fat 1.3g | Carbs 55g | Sugars 4.7g | Fibre 6.5g | Protein 14g | Salt 0.76g

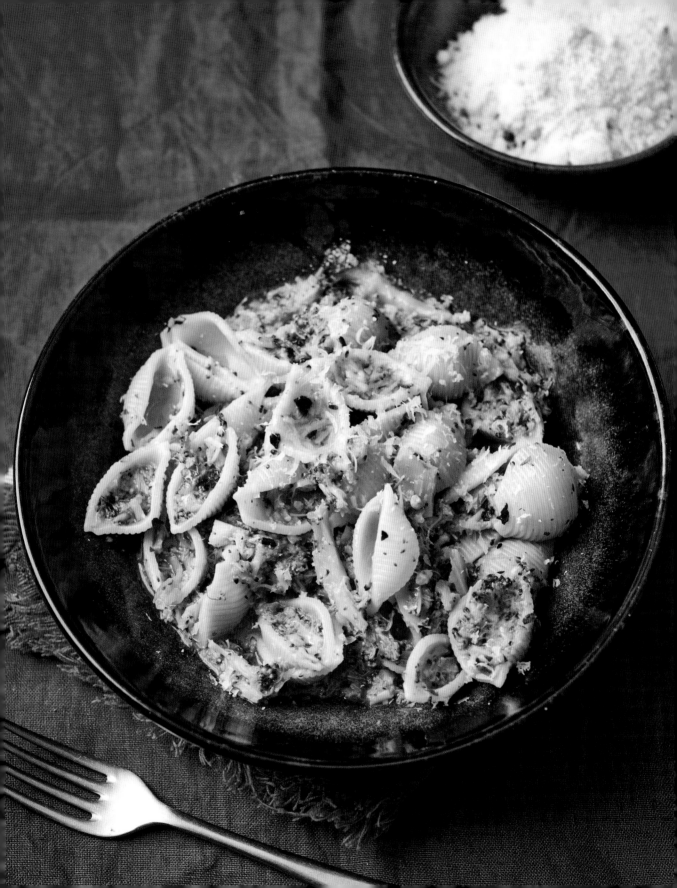

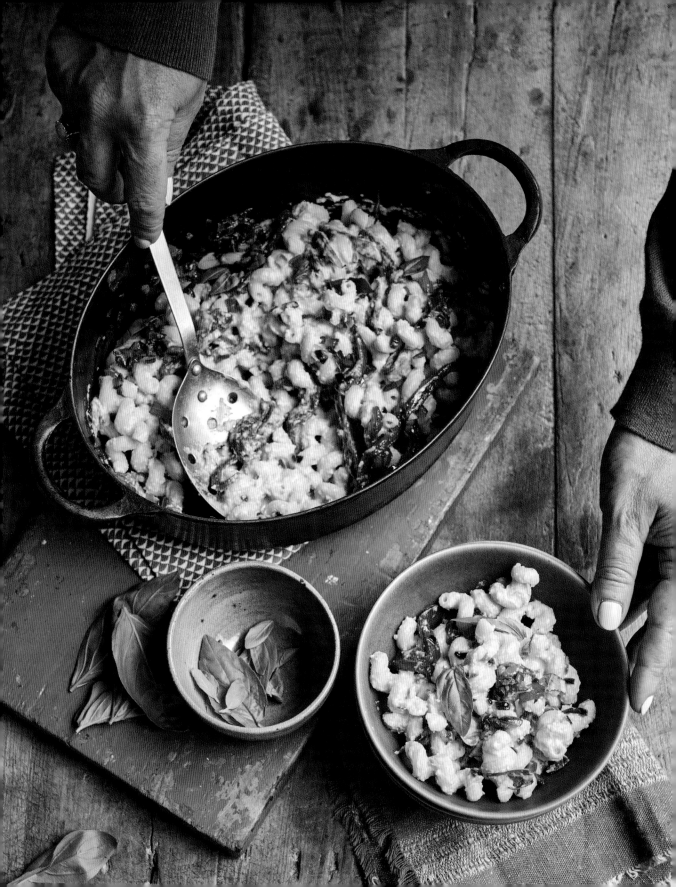

SERVES 2

HUMMUS PASTA

**Leftover hummus can make a fantastically easy pasta sauce
and is easy to customize with different vegetables and flavours.
You can make your own healthy hummus – see below, or try my Toasted
Walnut Hummus on page 193 – or just use a ready-made tub.**

PREP TIME: 5 MINUTES
COOK TIME: 12 MINUTES

150g (5½oz) spiral pasta (I use
   spirali or fusilli)
spray oil
1 small red onion, finely chopped
2 roasted red peppers in brine,
   from a jar, sliced
4 tablespoons hummus
small handful of basil leaves,
   shredded, plus extra leaves
   to serve
squeeze of lemon juice
salt and pepper, to taste

1. Cook the pasta in a large pan of boiling water for
   12 minutes
2. Meanwhile, spray a frying pan with oil and fry the onion
   gently, adding the roasted peppers for the last couple
   of minutes.
3. Drain the pasta, reserving a little of the cooking water,
   then return it to the empty pan. Stir the contents of the
   frying pan into the pasta with the hummus and basil,
   using a little of the cooking water to loosen it up and make
   sure it's not dry.
4. Season with the lemon juice, salt and pepper and serve
   scattered with basil leaves in warmed pasta bowls.

> **HOW TO MAKE YOUR OWN HUMMUS**
> You can save on calories by making your own basic hummus:
> Put a drained 400g (14oz) can of chickpeas into a mini
> chopper or food processor and add 1 garlic clove, the
> juice of ½ lemon, ½ teaspoon salt and 2 tablespoons
> fat-free Greek yogurt. Blend until smooth. You can
> customize the hummus with your favourite flavours
> such as chilli, smoked paprika or ground cumin.

PER SERVING: Calories 599 | Fat 16g | Sat Fat 1.8g | Carbs 91g | Sugars 20g | Fibre 10g | Protein 18g | Salt 0.9g

BLACK BEAN, CHIPOTLE & LIME SOUP

A delicious, warming Mexican-inspired soup with chipotle chilli, which has a smoky and sweet flavour. This is a filling soup served on its own, but I also love it with a handful of tortilla chips.

PREP TIME: 5 MINUTES
COOK TIME: 17 MINUTES

spray oil
1 celery stick, finely chopped
2 shallots, finely chopped
3 garlic cloves, crushed
½ teaspoon chipotle chilli flakes
½ teaspoon ground cumin
750ml (1 pint 5fl oz) hot
    vegetable stock
2 × 400g (14oz) cans of black
    beans, drained and rinsed
1 teaspoon dried oregano
small handful of coriander,
    plus extra leaves to serve
finely grated zest and juice of
    1 lime
salt and pepper, to taste
lime wedges, to serve (optional)

1. Spray a large saucepan with oil and fry the celery, shallots and garlic gently for 2 minutes.
2. Stir through the chipotle chilli flakes and ground cumin. Pour in the hot stock and add the black beans and oregano, then season with salt and pepper and simmer for 15 minutes.
3. Remove half the soup and use a stick blender to blend it with the coriander until smooth, then mix it back in with the unblended soup. (I pour mine into the jug that I used for the stock to blend it.)
4. Stir through the lime juice, then serve scattered with the lime zest and a few coriander leaves. Serve with extra lime wedges for squeezing over if you like.

NOTE Most supermarkets now have dried chipotle chilli flakes in their herb and spice selection, or sometimes you can find a chipotle chilli paste. If you can't get hold of chipotle chilli, then substitute regular crushed chillies plus ½ teaspoon smoked paprika.

PER SERVING: Calories 158 | Fat 1.1g | Sat Fat 0.1g | Carbs 20g | Sugars 9.1g | Fibre 12g | Protein 11g | Salt 2.2g

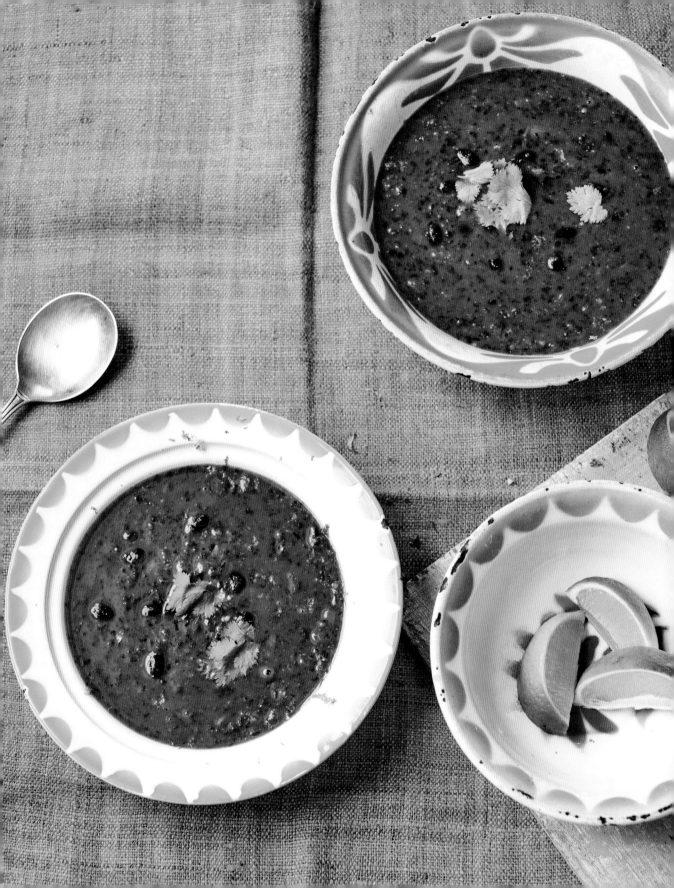

3 WAYS WITH STIR-FRY SAUCES

Stir-fries are one of the most versatile quick meals you can make because there are just so many ingredients you can throw in and it is a great way to use up leftovers.

1. Choose your protein. Stir-fries cook quickly, so use tender cuts of meat such as chicken breast or thigh fillet, pork tenderloin and beef fillet, or seafood such as salmon or prawns.
2. Choose your vegetables. Firm vegetables such as onions, carrots, baby corn and broccoli will take longer to cook. Quick-cooking options include spring onions, spinach, pak choi, peppers, bean sprouts, mushrooms, courgette and sugarsnap peas.

To cook a stir-fry, start by frying the protein. If using meat, fry it in spray oil until no pink remains before starting to add the vegetables. Add the longer-cooking vegetables first and fry for a few minutes, before adding the quicker-cooking vegetables. If using salmon or prawns, add them at the same time as the quicker-cooking vegetables. Stir-fry everything for 2–3 minutes until nearly cooked, then add the stir-fry sauce, stirring it in and cooking for 2–3 minutes. Serve over rice or noodles.

SERVES 4

HONEY SRIRACHA

Spicy and sweet, this simple sauce is a quick way to make a great-tasting stir-fry.

PREP TIME: 1 MINUTE

COOK TIME: NONE

2 tablespoons sriracha
2 tablespoons honey
4 tablespoons dark soy sauce
4 garlic cloves, crushed
5cm (2 inch) piece of fresh root
   ginger, peeled and finely grated

1. Simply mix the ingredients together in a small bowl and stir-fry into your protein and vegetables when needed (see method above).

PER SERVING: Calories 61 | Fat 0g | Sat Fat 0g | Carbs 15g | Sugars 14g | Fibre 0g | Protein 0.5g | Salt 2.5g

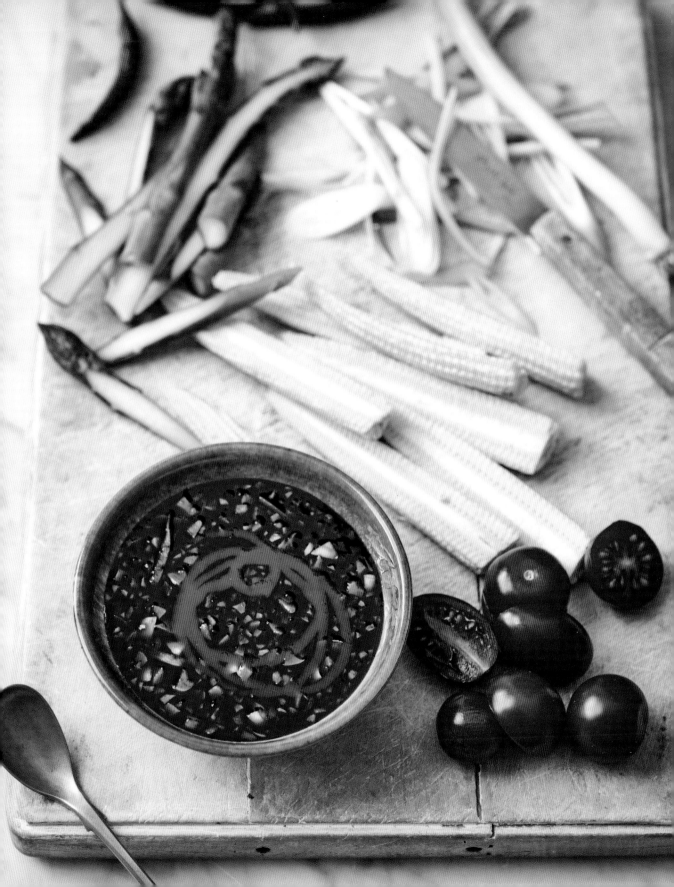

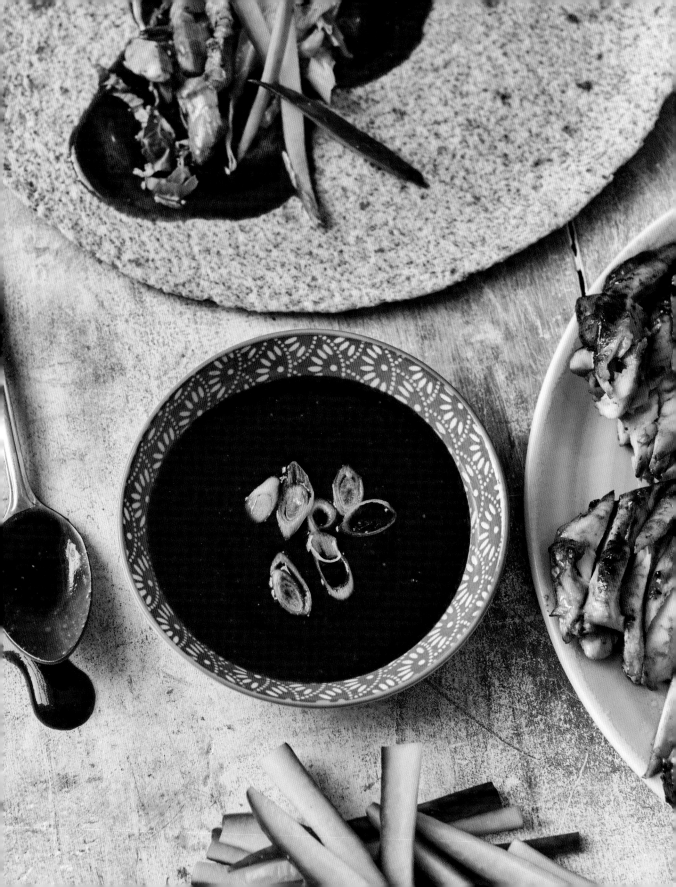

HOISIN SAUCE

**Hoisin is a strong, salty, umami sauce with a hint of sweet,
and is so flavoursome that it can jazz up most stir-fries.
Try this with my Hoisin Chicken Wraps (see page 155).**

PREP TIME: 2 MINUTES
COOK TIME: 3 MINUTES

4 tablespoons light soy sauce
2 tablespoons smooth peanut
  butter
2 tablespoons honey
2 tablespoons rice vinegar
½ teaspoon Chinese five spice
1 teaspoon cornflour

1. Put all the ingredients, except the cornflour, in a small pan and heat through for 2 minutes, stirring constantly to form a smooth sauce.
2. Put the cornflour into a small bowl or cup and mix it with a splash of cold water into a smooth liquid, then pour into the sauce and stir for a minute or so until the sauce thickens.
3. Allow the sauce to cool, then serve cold as a condiment or use in a stir-fry (see method on page 58). Store in an airtight container in the refrigerator. It will keep for up to 2 weeks.

PER SERVING: Calories 108 | Fat 4.8g | Sat Fat 1.2g | Carbs 13g | Sugars 11g | Fibre 0.7g | Protein 2.6g | Salt 1.9g

LEMON SESAME SAUCE

A bright lemony stir-fry sauce, which will go down a treat with the whole family.

PREP TIME: 2 MINUTES
COOK TIME: NONE

1 teaspoon cornflour
finely grated zest and juice of
    1 lemon
1 teaspoon toasted sesame oil
100ml (3½fl oz) chicken stock
2 garlic cloves, crushed
2 tablespoons light soy sauce
1 teaspoon brown sugar
1 teaspoon sesame seeds

1. Dissolve the cornflour in the lemon juice, then stir in all the remaining ingredients apart from the sesame seeds.
2. When you cook the sauce with the vegetables (see method on page 58), keep stirring it for 2–3 minutes until the sauce slightly thickens and coats the other ingredients.
3. Scatter over the sesame seeds to serve.

PER SERVING: Calories 54 | Fat 1.9g | Sat Fat 0.3g | Carbs 7g | Sugars 5.1g | Fibre 0.5g | Protein 1g | Salt 1.7g

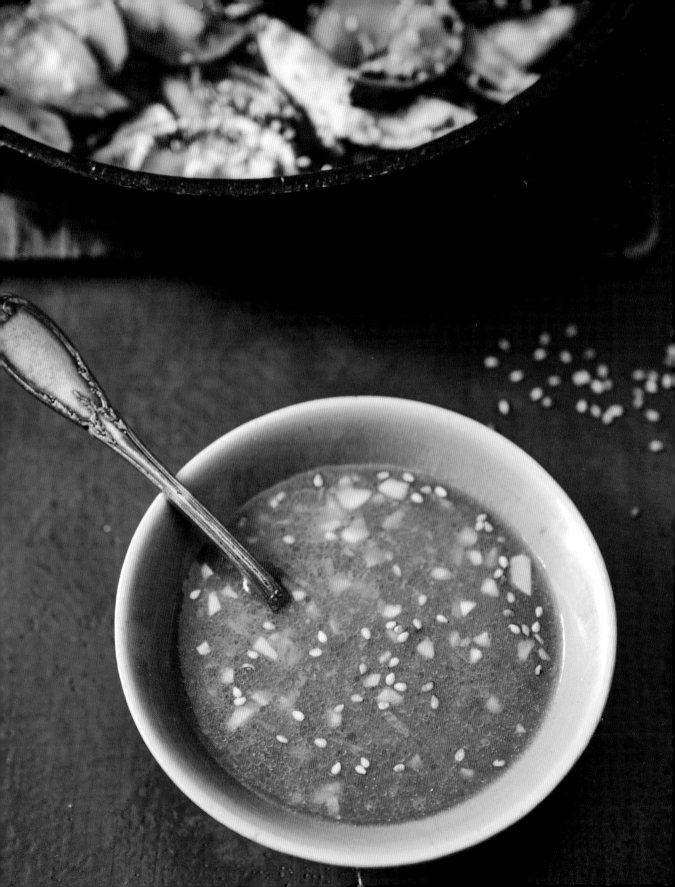

CHAPTER 3

MIDWEEK WINNERS

LIGHT LEMON, SMOKED SALMON & PEA SPAGHETTI

A light and summery pasta dish; the sauce is ready in the time it takes the pasta to cook.

PREP TIME: 3 MINUTES
COOK TIME: 12 MINUTES

350g (12oz) spaghetti
250g (9oz) frozen peas
finely grated zest and juice of
   1 lemon
4 tablespoons half-fat crème
   fraîche
15g (½oz) Parmesan cheese,
   finely grated
180g (6oz) smoked salmon, cut
   into strips
salt and pepper, to taste
handful of parsley leaves,
   to serve

1. Cook the spaghetti in a large pan of boiling water. After 7 minutes, add the frozen peas to cook with the spaghetti.

2. When the spaghetti is cooked, drain it, reserving a little of the cooking water.

3. Put the drained spaghetti back into the pan and add the lemon juice, crème fraîche, Parmesan, smoked salmon and salt and pepper, plus a little of the reserved pasta water. Stir everything together thoroughly.

4. Divide between 4 warmed plates or bowls and scatter with the lemon zest, parsley and freshly ground black pepper.

NOTE If you want to increase the vegetables in this, add 125g (4½oz) asparagus spears, woody ends trimmed away and sliced into 1cm (½ inch) lengths, to cook with the spaghetti at the same time as the peas.

PER SERVING: Calories 520 | Fat 13g | Sat Fat 5.7g | Carbs 69g | Sugars 7.5g | Fibre 6.9g | Protein 27g | Salt 1.7g

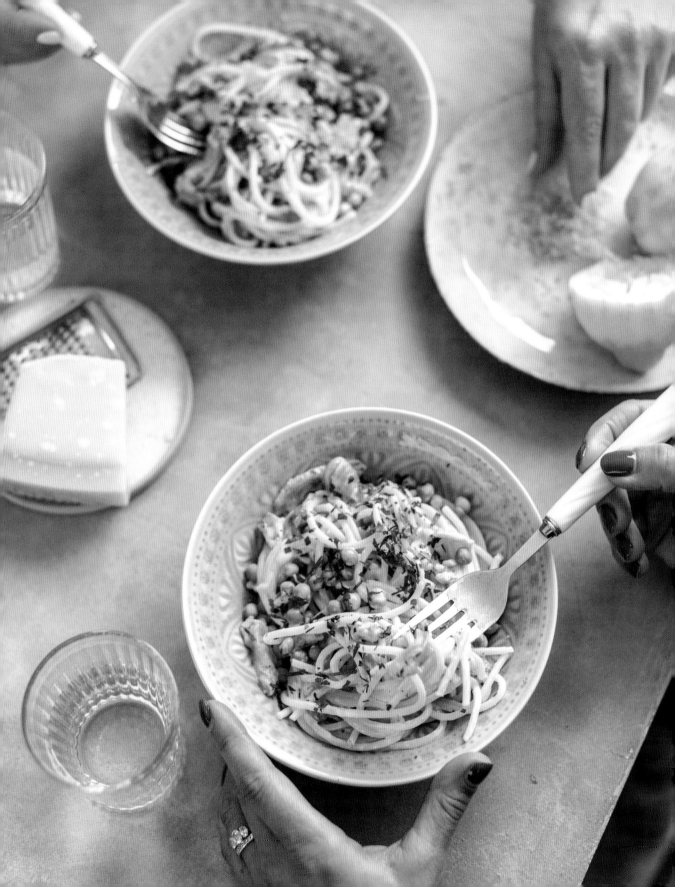

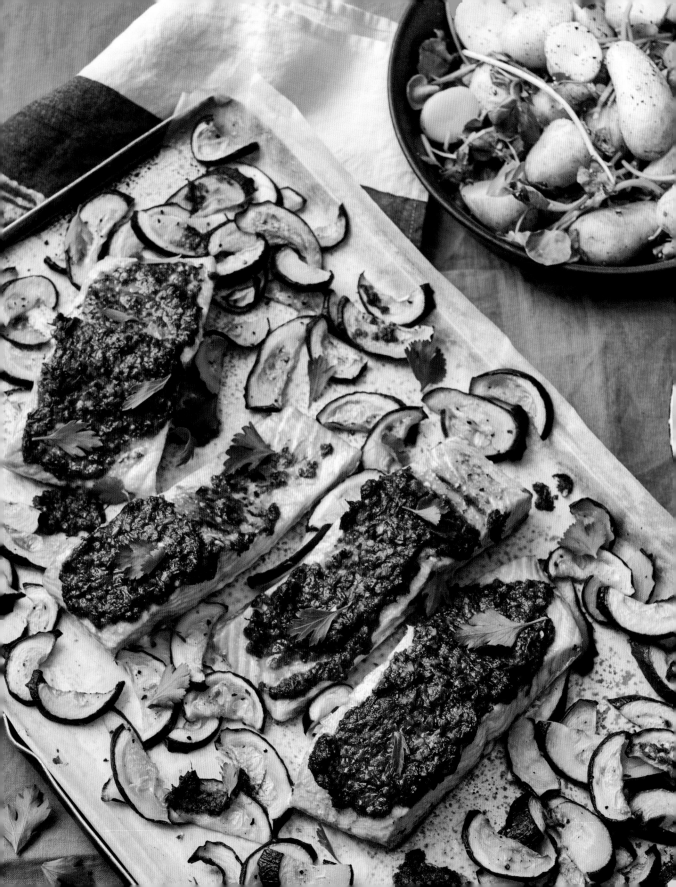

CHERMOULA BAKED SALMON

WITH BABY NEW POTATOES & COURGETTES

You can find pre-made chermoula paste in bigger supermarkets and it's a fantastic ingredient for adding quick flavour to meals. If you can't get hold of it, then you can easily make your own in a flash (see page 202).

PREP TIME: 5 MINUTES

COOK TIME: 22 MINUTES

2 courgettes (total weight about 500g / 1lb 2oz), trimmed, halved lengthways, then sliced 1cm (½ inch) thick

spray oil

4 salmon fillets

2 tablespoons chermoula (for homemade, see page 202)

500g (1lb 2oz) baby new potatoes, cut in half, depending on size

2 mint sprigs

juice of 1 lemon

1 teaspoon coarse salt

salt and pepper, to taste

80g (2¾oz) watercress, or other salad leaves of your choice, to serve

1. Preheat the oven to 220°C/200°C fan (425°F), Gas Mark 7.
2. Place the sliced courgettes on a baking tray lined with nonstick baking paper, season them, spray lightly with oil and bake for 10 minutes.
3. Remove the courgettes from the oven, use a spatula to move them to the edges of the tray and lie the salmon fillets in the centre, skin-side down.
4. Spread the chermoula paste evenly over the top of the salmon fillets and spray with a little oil. Put the tray back in the oven for 12 minutes.
5. Meanwhile, place the new potatoes into a large pan of boiling water with the mint sprigs and simmer for 15 minutes until tender.
6. Drain the potatoes, then toss them with the lemon juice, coarse salt and watercress.
7. Serve the potatoes and watercress with the salmon and courgettes or with other salad leaves on the side.

NOTE If you can't source chermoula, swap it out for another ready-made paste, any of my Pesto recipes (see pages 128–133) or tapenade. If you are able to get hold of watercress, this will wilt slightly when you toss it with the potatoes. This would also work well with spinach leaves. If you use other fresh salad leaves, just serve them on the side to maintain their freshness.

PER SERVING: Calories 404 | Fat 17g | Sat Fat 2.4g | Carbs 21g | Sugars 4.3g | Fibre 5.7g | Protein 3g | Salt 1.5g

SARAH'S STICKY SALMON
WITH BROCCOLI

My friend Sarah shared this recipe with me; it was something she had thrown together in a rush on a weeknight and was a hit with the whole family. Garlic and ginger pastes are really handy to have in the refrigerator for those days when you just don't have time for prepping and chopping. If you wish, you could serve this with noodles or rice.

PREP TIME: 5 MINUTES
COOK TIME: 17 MINUTES

2 heads of broccoli, broken into florets, each floret sliced in half
1 teaspoon toasted sesame oil
2 tablespoons dark soy sauce
2 tablespoons honey
1 teaspoon garlic paste
1 teaspoon ginger paste
4 salmon fillets
4 spring onions, finely sliced, to serve

1. Preheat the oven to 220°C/ 200°C fan (425°F), Gas Mark 7.
2. Place the broccoli florets into a baking dish, drizzle over the sesame oil and toss the broccoli around to coat it in the oil. Pop into the oven and bake for 5 minutes.
3. Meanwhile, make up the sauce in a small bowl by mixing together the soy sauce, honey, garlic and ginger.
4. After 5 minutes, remove the broccoli from the oven and give it a good stir around in the dish. Place the salmon fillets, skin side down, in the baking dish and spoon the sauce over each fillet, drizzling any remaining sauce over the broccoli.
5. Place in the oven and cook for 12 minutes.
6. Serve, removing the skin from the salmon fillets, if you like, then scattering with the spring onions.

NOTE You can add extra vegetables to the tray to cook if you wish at the same time as the broccoli. Onion wedges, pepper strips, cauliflower florets, green beans and asparagus spears all work well.

PER SERVING: Calories 390 | Fat 18g | Sat Fat 2.4g | Carbs 16g | Sugars 13g | Fibre 5.3g | Protein 38g | Salt 1.8g

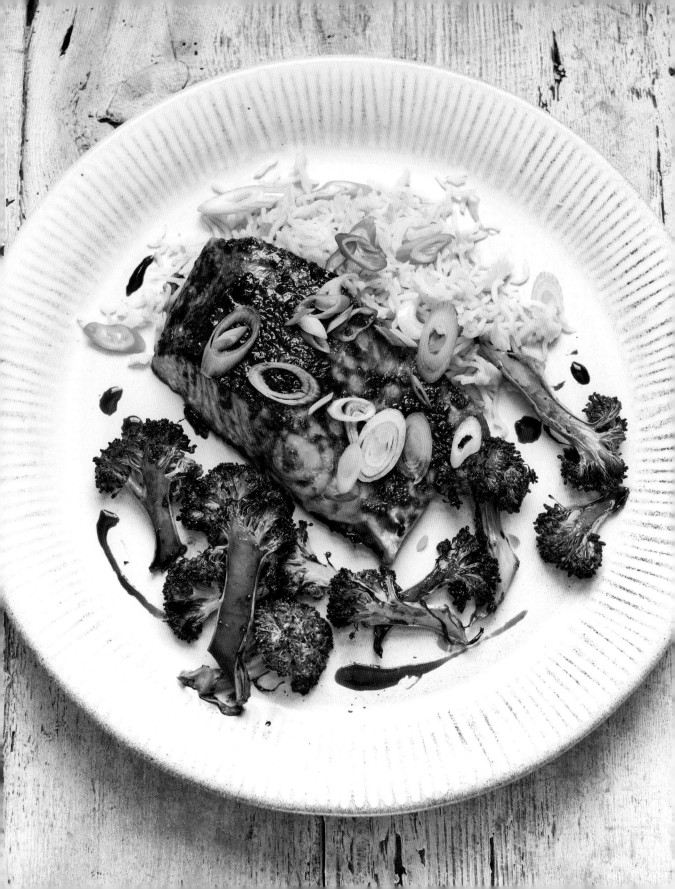

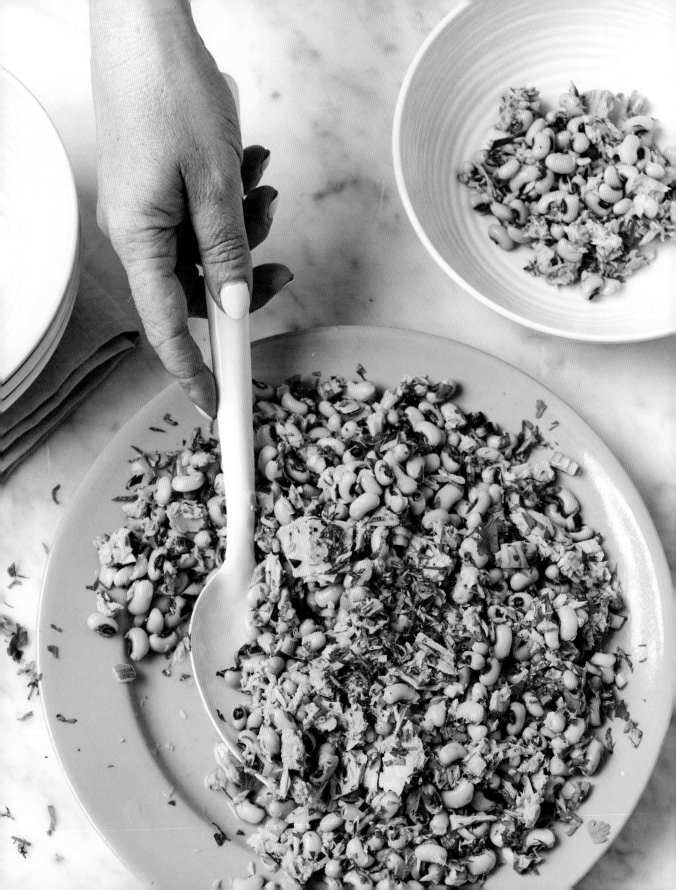

TUNA & BLACK-EYED BEAN SALAD

This is a great, filling salad, using just a few store-cupboard staples. Keep it in the refrigerator for a quick and easy lunch, or make a big batch to take along to summer barbecues. I usually serve it with wholemeal pitta and salad leaves.

PREP TIME: 5 MINUTES
COOK TIME: NONE

2 × 400g (14oz) cans of black-eyed beans, drained and rinsed
1 small red onion, very finely chopped
large handful of parsley leaves, finely chopped
2 × 145g (5¼oz) cans of tuna in spring water, drained
salt and pepper, to taste

FOR THE VINAIGRETTE
3 tablespoons rice vinegar
2 teaspoons Dijon mustard
1 garlic clove, crushed

1. Put the black-eyed beans in a large bowl with the onion, parsley and salt and pepper and mix thoroughly.
2. Make the vinaigrette by whisking together all the ingredients in a small bowl with a fork, then add the tuna and vinaigrette to the large bowl and season well. Mix together carefully, without mashing up the tuna.

NOTE You can add extras to this if you have time for more chopping! Some nice additions are finely chopped sweet pepper, peeled, pitted and chopped avocado, chopped rocket, cucumber, baby tomatoes... this salad is a great way to have a clear-out of any ingredients in the refrigerator that need using up!

PER SERVING: Calories 202 | Fat 1.7g | Sat Fat 0.3g | Carbs 18g | Sugars 7.4g | Fibre 11g | Protein 22g | Salt 1.3g

TUNA & OLIVE RIGATONI

A simple and delicious pasta dish with some of the key flavours of a puttanesca, using canned tuna for an easy store-cupboard meal.

PREP TIME: 5 MINUTES
COOK TIME: 17 MINUTES

1 teaspoon olive oil
2 shallots, finely sliced
1 bird's eye chilli, deseeded and
   finely chopped
3 garlic cloves, crushed
400g (14oz) can of chopped
   tomatoes
400g (14oz) rigatoni pasta
1 tablespoon tomato purée
50g (1¾oz) pitted black olives,
   sliced
1 teaspoon balsamic vinegar
2 teaspoons dried oregano
leaves from 1 rosemary sprig,
   finely chopped
145g (5¼oz) can of tuna in
   spring water, drained
salt and pepper, to taste

TO SERVE
handful of parsley leaves,
   finely chopped
Parmesan cheese, finely grated

1. Heat the oil in a sauté pan and gently fry the shallots for 3 minutes, then stir through the chilli and garlic. Pour in the can of chopped tomatoes and stir.
2. Cook the pasta in a large pan of boiling water and set a timer for 12 minutes.
3. While the pasta is cooking, add the tomato purée to the shallot mixture with the olives, balsamic vinegar, oregano and rosemary and season with salt and pepper. Stir and leave to simmer gently, stirring occasionally. As the tomatoes soften, you can help to break them down with a wooden spoon.
4. Drain the pasta, reserving a little of the cooking water.
5. Stir the tuna through the tomato sauce, add a little bit of pasta water and leave it on the heat for a couple more minutes, allowing the tuna to heat through.
6. Stir the rigatoni through the sauce and serve, scattered with parsley and sprinkled with Parmesan.

NOTE For a vegetarian version, simply leave out the tuna and Parmesan (or use Parmesan-style vegetarian cheese) and double the amount of olives.

PER SERVING: Calories 451 | Fat 5.4g | Sat Fat 0.7g | Carbs 75g | Sugars 9.8g | Fibre 7.4g | Protein 20g | Salt 0.65g

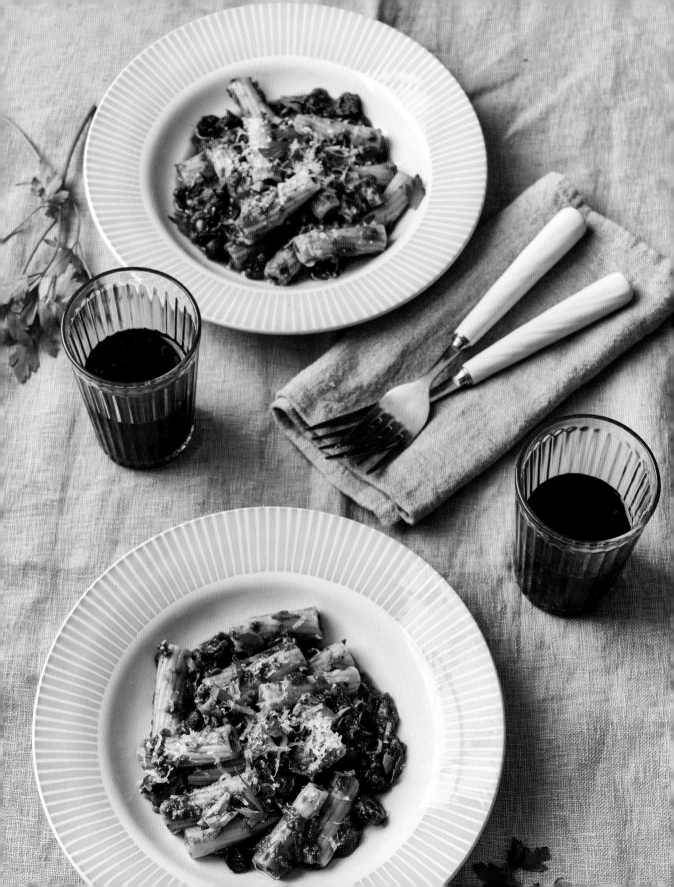

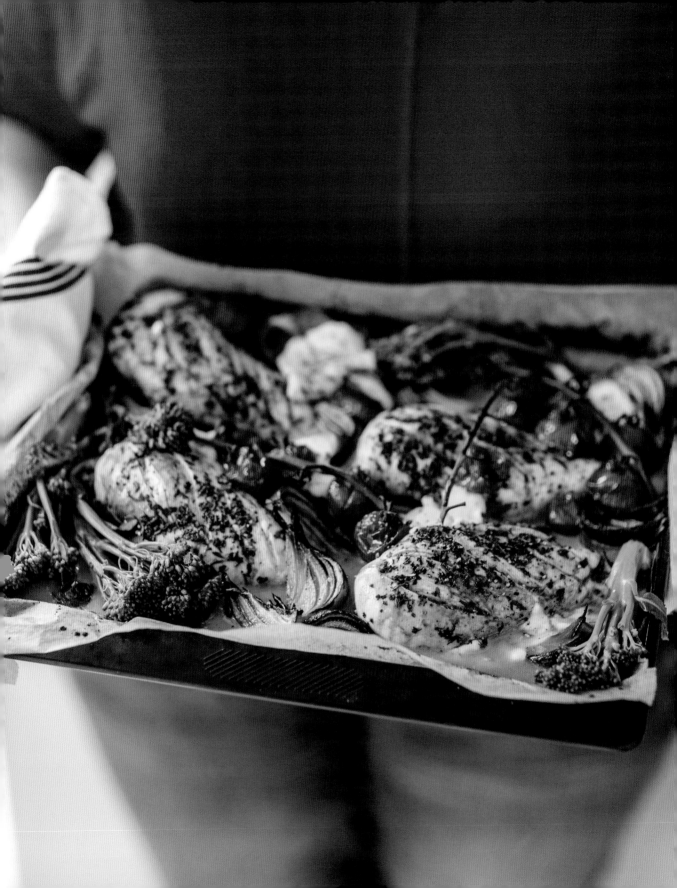

BALSAMIC CHICKEN BAKE
WITH TENDERSTEM BROCCOLI

Succulent chicken breasts served over roasted tomatoes in a tangy balsamic sauce, finished off with oozing, bubbling mozzarella. Simple ingredients, maximum flavour.

PREP TIME: 5 MINUTES
COOK TIME: 24 MINUTES

2 tablespoons balsamic vinegar
1 tablespoon honey
1 teaspoon dried oregano, plus a
    pinch to serve
1 teaspoon dried basil
4 skinless chicken breasts
500g (1lb 2oz) cherry tomatoes
    on the vine, or baby plum
    tomatoes
2 red onions, cut into wedges
spray oil
125g (4½oz) mozzarella cheese,
    torn into pieces
200g (7oz) Tenderstem broccoli
salt and pepper, to taste

1. Preheat the oven to 240°C/220°C fan (475°F), Gas Mark 9.
2. In a shallow bowl, make up a sauce with the balsamic vinegar, honey, oregano and basil.
3. With a sharp knife, score each chicken breast all the way across on the diagonal, cutting about three-quarters of the way down through the breast, and spacing the cuts about 1cm (½ inch) apart. This will help the chicken to cook evenly all the way through.
4. Place the chicken breasts, cut side up, into a baking dish and arrange the tomatoes and onions around them. Pour over the sauce, season with salt and pepper and spray everything lightly with oil.
5. Place in the oven and bake for 15 minutes. Remove from the oven, arrange the mozzarella over the chicken and bake for a further 5 minutes to melt the cheese. Remove from the oven and set aside while you cook the broccoli.
6. Cook the broccoli in a pan of simmering water for 4 minutes, then drain.
7. Serve the chicken and tomatoes, with their juices, in 4 warmed pasta bowls, with the broccoli on the side and a pinch of dried oregano scattered over the top.

> **A TIME-SAVING TIP**
> If you ever have odd leftover chicken breasts, cut them into chunks before freezing so that they defrost more quickly and are ready to go for quick stir-fries or curries.

PER SERVING: Calories 344 | Fat 10g | Sat Fat 5.2g | Carbs 16g | Sugars 14g | Fibre 3.6g | Protein 44g | Salt 0.9g

HEARTY CHICKEN, BACON & AVOCADO SALAD

If I'm having a salad as my main meal, then I want to make sure it is really going to fill me up! This is a simple recipe with few ingredients, but it's filling, satisfying and delicious.

PREP TIME: 5 MINUTES
COOK TIME: 15 MINUTES

spray oil
1 chicken breast, sliced in half
   horizontally
2 bacon medallions
100g (3½oz) mixed salad leaves
8 baby tomatoes, quartered
1 avocado, peeled, pitted and
   chopped
1 tablespoon sunflower seeds
salt and pepper, to taste

FOR THE VINAIGRETTE
2 tablespoons red wine vinegar
1 garlic clove, crushed
1 teaspoon Dijon mustard
1 teaspoon Italian-style mixed
   dried herbs

1. Spray a large frying pan with oil and fry the chicken breast halves side by side for 5 minutes. Add the bacon medallions and fry them together with the chicken for another 10 minutes, flipping over every now and again.

2. Once the chicken has fried for 15 minutes and you have checked that it is cooked through (see page 109), season it with salt and pepper and set it aside to rest with the bacon while you prepare the rest of the salad.

3. To make the dressing, combine the red wine vinegar, garlic, mustard, dried herbs and a little salt and pepper. I find it easiest to put all the ingredients into a clean jam jar and shake them together, but you could put them in a small bowl and just whisk them together using a fork.

4. Split the salad leaves between 2 bowls, then scatter in the tomatoes and avocado.

5. Use a sharp knife to slice the chicken and cut the bacon into thin strips, then divide these between the 2 bowls.

6. Drizzle the vinaigrette over each salad, then top with the sunflower seeds. Serve immediately.

PER SERVING: Calories 312 | Fat 20g | Sat Fat 3.9g | Carbs 6.9g | Sugars 3.8g | Fibre 5.2g | Protein 23g | Salt 1.9g

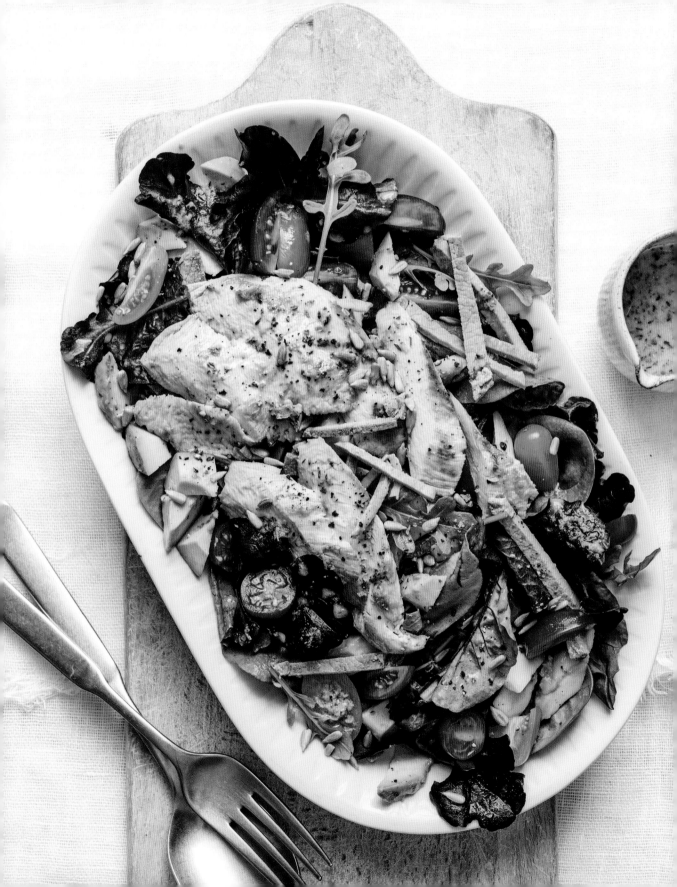

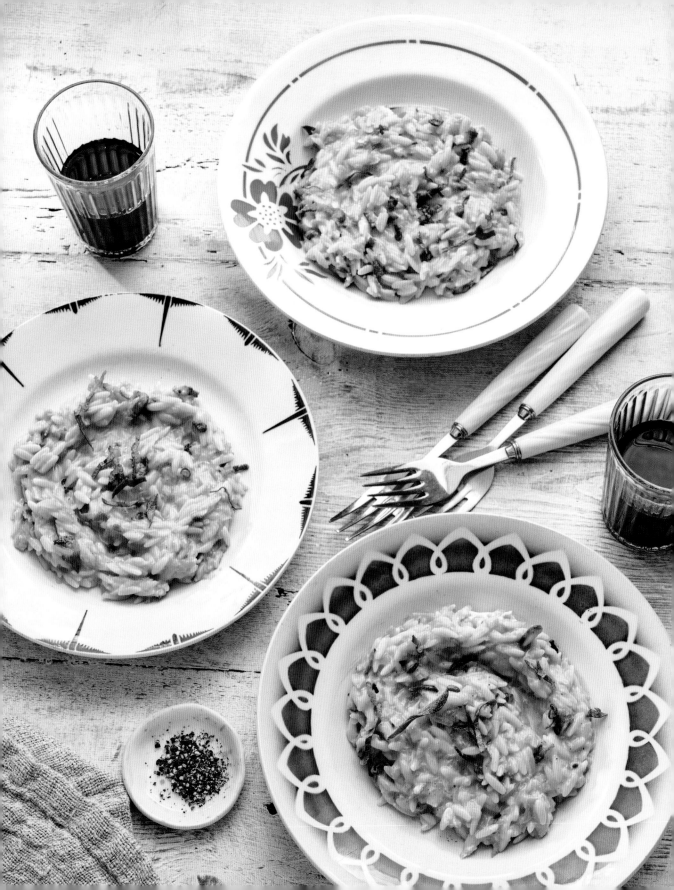

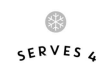

CREAMY BACON, SAGE & SQUASH ORZOTTO

Orzo makes a brilliant quick meal that resembles a risotto but with much less room for error. Grating butternut squash allows it to cook quickly and makes a creamy sauce. I like to serve this with steamed asparagus, because a vegetable side dish with a bit of a bite really complements the meal. I sometimes freeze pasta dishes containing orzo, macaroni and couscous, but the texture may differ from when it is freshly cooked.

PREP TIME: 5 MINUTES
COOK TIME: 25 MINUTES

4 smoked streaky bacon rashers, finely sliced
1 onion, finely chopped
3 garlic cloves, crushed
about 14 sage leaves, finely sliced
200g (7oz) orzo pasta
750ml (1 pint 5fl oz) hot chicken stock
200g (7oz) butternut squash, grated (see note)
75g (2¾oz) reduced-fat cream cheese
salt and pepper, to taste

1. Stir-fry the bacon, onion, garlic and sage over a medium heat for 5 minutes; there's no need for oil, as the fat from the bacon will be enough.
2. Stir through the orzo, then pour in the hot stock. Grate in the butternut squash. Bring up to a fast simmer for 15–20 minutes, stirring regularly to prevent sticking. If the orzotto looks like it is drying out too much, just add a little extra hot water. After 15 minutes, try a little bit of the orzo to see if it is cooked though; if not, keep simmering for a minute or so and then test again.
3. When the orzo is cooked, turn off the heat, season with salt and pepper and stir through the cream cheese until it's fully combined.

NOTE To save on prep time for this meal, I grate the butternut squash directly into the pan as the orzo cooks: I cut off the stalk end of a butternut squash just at the point where it becomes bulbous. This top section is usually solid with no cavity or seeds. I use a vegetable peeler to peel the skin off and it is then easy to grate into the pan.

Note that different brands of orzo can differ in size and may take longer to cook than others. Most cook in 15–20 minutes.

PER SERVING: Calories 312 | Fat 9.1g | Sat Fat 3.2g | Carbs 42g | Sugars 6.9g | Fibre 4.4g | Protein 13g | Salt 3.3g

BAKED RICOTTA, CHORIZO & SPINACH SPAGHETTI

Baked ricotta is a perfect consistency to stir through cooked pasta, while a few simple added ingredients mean maximum flavour for minimum effort. Simply throw everything for the sauce into a tray with the cheese and bake them before stirring in the cooked pasta.

PREP TIME: 8 MINUTES
COOK TIME: 20 MINUTES

250g (9oz) ricotta cheese
1 red onion, cut into wedges
2 garlic cloves, finely sliced
325g (11½oz) cherry tomatoes, halved
40g (1½oz) chorizo, finely chopped
1 teaspoon dried oregano
spray oil
300g (10½oz) spaghetti
2 large handfuls of baby spinach leaves, roughly sliced
salt and pepper, to taste

1. Preheat the oven to 220°C/200°C fan (425°F), Gas Mark 7. Find a medium-large baking dish about 26 × 22cm (10½ × 8½ inches).
2. Place the ricotta in the middle of the dish, then scatter the onion, garlic, tomatoes and chorizo all around the edge. Scatter the oregano over and season with salt and pepper.
3. Spray the vegetables lightly with oil and bake for 20 minutes.
4. Meanwhile, cook the spaghetti according to the packet instructions, then drain it, reserving a little of the cooking water. Mix the spinach through the cooked spaghetti in the colander.
5. Remove the dish from the oven and tip in the spaghetti and spinach. Thoroughly mix everything together so that the cheese coats the strands of spaghetti and the vegetables have mixed in evenly. If you need to loosen up the sauce, just mix in a little of the pasta cooking water.

NOTE This method will work with other types of cheese, including feta, cream cheese, or garlic and herb roulé. You can also mix it up by trying different types of vegetables such as courgettes, peppers and mushrooms, or different herbs such as basil, parsley or mixed herbs. For a vegetarian version, just omit the chorizo and ensure that your chosen cheese is suitable for vegetarians.

PER SERVING: Calories 444 | Fat 13g | Sat Fat 6.2g | Carbs 59g | Sugars 7.7g | Fibre 4.4g | Protein 19g | Salt 0.6g

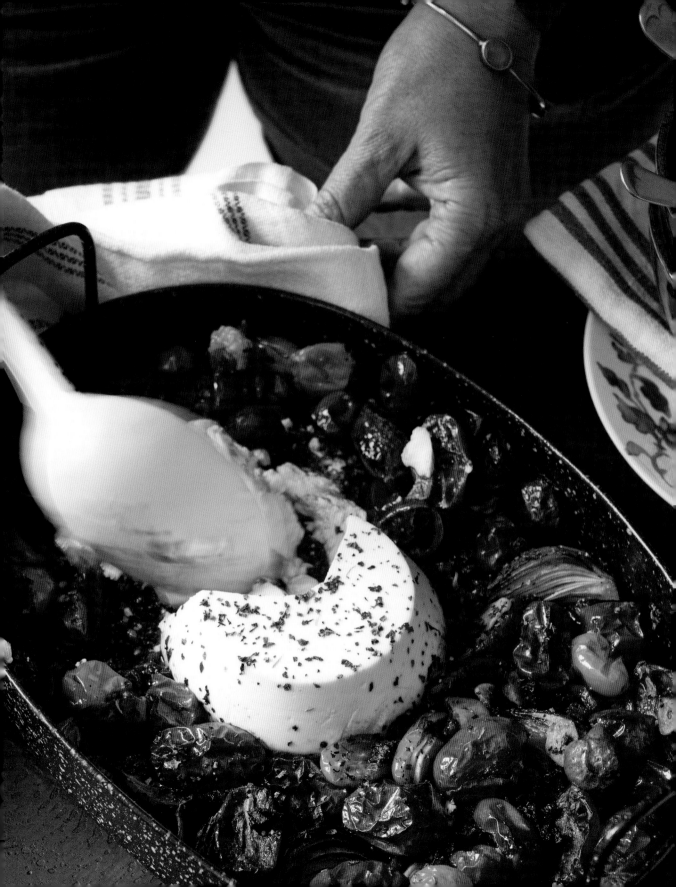

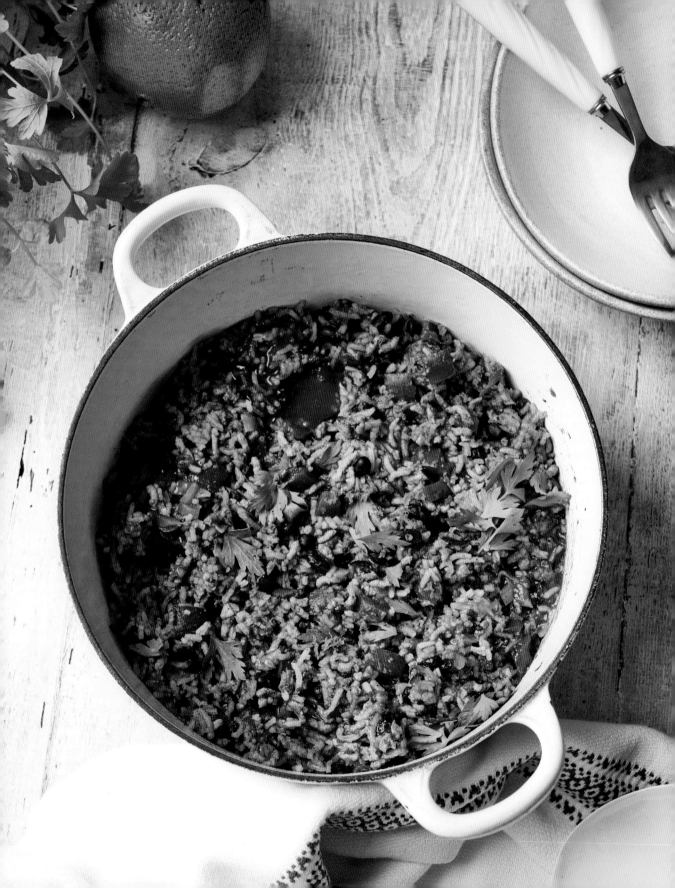

LIGHTLY SPICED BLACK BEAN, PORK & ORANGE STEW

Inspired by Brazilian flavours, this one-pot rice dish is great on its own or with green veg such as broccoli, green beans or asparagus.

PREP TIME: 5 MINUTES

COOK TIME: 25 MINUTES

spray oil

1 onion, finely chopped

500g (1lb 2oz) lean minced pork (5 per cent fat)

3 garlic cloves, crushed

1 red pepper, deseeded and finely chopped

1 teaspoon ground cumin

1 teaspoon ground coriander

½ teaspoon ground allspice

160g (5¾oz) white long grain rice

500ml (18fl oz) hot chicken stock

400g (14oz) can of chopped tomatoes

400g (14oz) can of black beans, drained and rinsed

finely grated zest and juice of 1 orange

1 tablespoon dried oregano

salt and pepper, to taste

TO SERVE

handful of chopped parsley

zest of ½ orange

1. Spray a large, deep pan with oil and fry the onion, pork and garlic for 5 minutes, stirring and breaking up the clumps of meat as it cooks.
2. Stir in the pepper, then the spices. Stir in the rice, then pour in the hot stock and chopped tomatoes and bring to the boil.
3. Add the black beans, orange zest and juice, oregano and salt and pepper, then reduce the heat so the pot is simmering and cook for 20 minutes, stirring occasionally.
4. After 20 minutes, check the rice to see if it is cooked (it should not be chalky). If it's still not quite cooked then give it a couple of extra minutes; you can add a little boiling water if it looks like it needs a bit more liquid.
5. Serve scattered with the parsley and finely grate over more orange zest to serve.

> **GROW YOUR OWN**
> Parsley is one of the easiest herbs to grow at home. A sunny windowsill is an ideal spot. You can extend the life of a supermarket herb plant by repotting it. You will need some multipurpose compost and a couple of larger plant pots to allow the roots room to grow (make sure there are drainage holes at the bottom). Most herb pots can be gently split into 2–3 clumps and repotted to give them a whole new lease of life. Just water regularly.

PER SERVING: Calories 458 | Fat 8.2g | Sat Fat 2.5g | Carbs 52g | Sugars 15g | Fibre 9.1g | Protein 38g | Salt 2.9g

PORK, GINGER & LIME MEATBALLS

Bright, zesty flavour is packed into these quick meatballs.

PREP TIME: 10 MINUTES
COOK TIME: 12 MINUTES

500g (1lb 2oz) lean minced pork
    (5 per cent fat)
5cm (2 inch) piece of fresh root
    ginger, peeled and finely grated
2 garlic cloves, crushed
2 spring onions, finely chopped
1 green chilli, deseeded and
    finely chopped
finely grated zest and juice of
    1 lime, plus extra lime wedges
    to serve
1 tablespoon fish sauce
300g (10½oz) jasmine rice
spray oil
1 courgette, cut in half lengthways
    then finely sliced
2 tablespoons dark soy sauce
1 tablespoon sweet chilli sauce
1 carrot, cut into matchsticks
salt, to taste
coriander leaves, to serve

1. In a large bowl, mix together the pork, ginger, garlic, spring onions, chilli, lime zest and juice, fish sauce and a pinch of salt.
2. Roll the mixture into small, bite-sized meatballs; you should get about 30.
3. Cook the rice according to the packet instructions (usually around 12 minutes).
4. Meanwhile, spray a sauté pan with spray oil and fry the meatballs for 10 minutes, stirring occasionally.
5. Add the courgette, soy sauce and sweet chilli sauce to the meatball pan and stir-fry for 2 minutes.
6. Serve the rice, then top with the raw carrot, meatballs and courgette mixture. Scatter with coriander leaves and serve with lime wedges. The meatballs can be frozen, but not the rice.

TIPS FOR STORING FRESH ROOT GINGER
You can freeze fresh ginger so you always have it readily available and never let it go to waste. If you have a big root, cut it into smaller pieces – most of my recipes require a 2cm (¾ inch) or 5cm (2 inch) piece. Simply put the ginger into a sealable freezer bag or freezer-safe container and label it so that you remember what's in there. You can peel and grate it from frozen, which will work in lots of recipes. If you need sliced ginger for recipes, allow it to defrost before trying to slice it.

PER SERVING: Calories 477 | Fat 7.1g | Sat Fat 2.4g | Carbs 67g | Sugars 7.5g | Fibre 2.3g | Protein 34g | Salt 2.8g

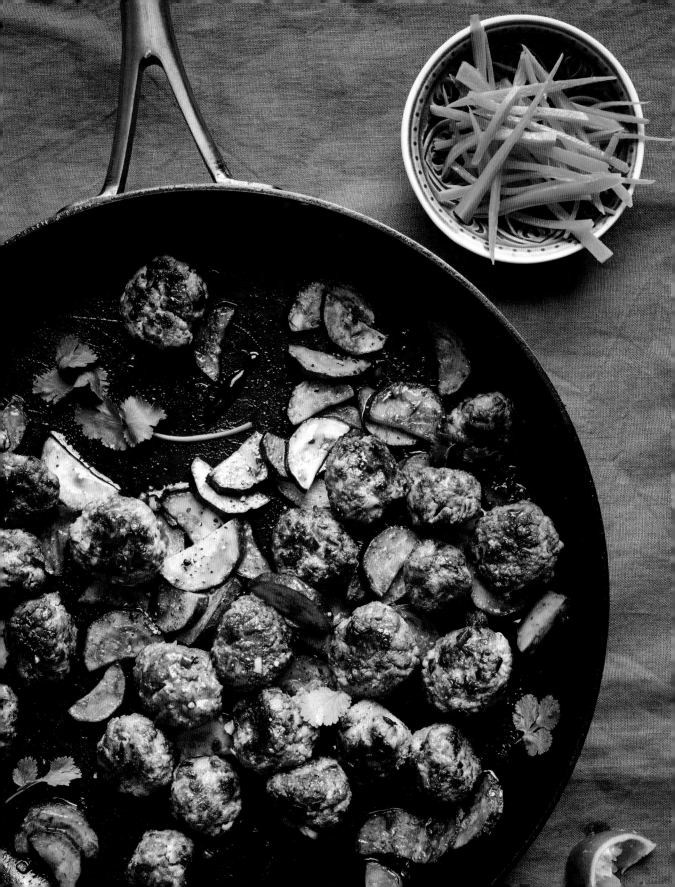

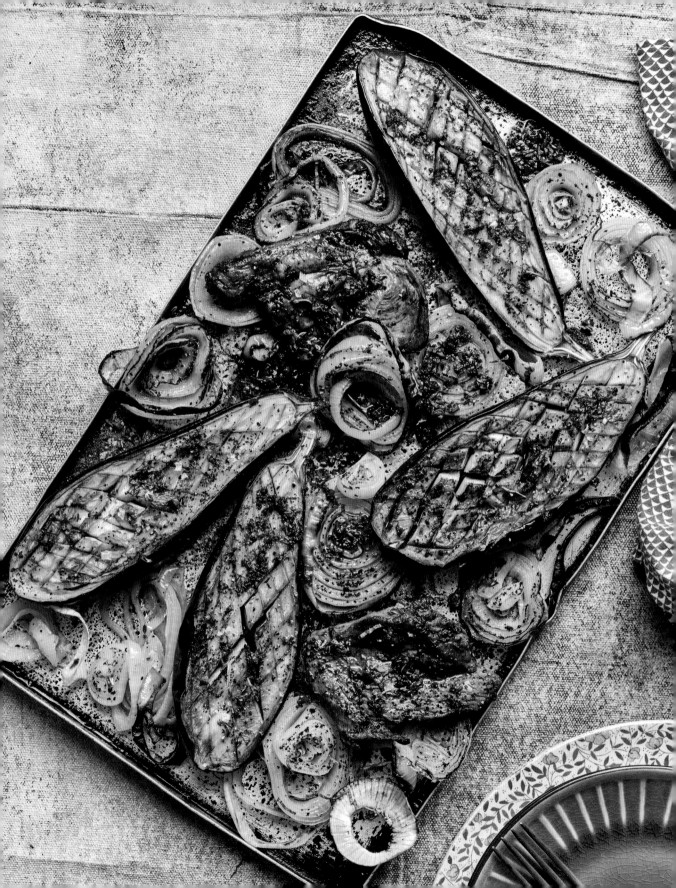

GRILLED LAMB & AUBERGINE

WITH HOT MINT SAUCE

Most of the work for this meal is done by a hot grill. Buttery soft grilled aubergine and sweet grilled onions are the ideal side dish for simple lamb steaks. A hot mint sauce provides a burst of mouth-watering flavour.

PREP TIME: 10 MINUTES
COOK TIME: 14 MINUTES

2 lamb leg steaks
2 aubergines, halved lengthways
   and flesh scored diagonally
   in a criss-cross pattern (be
   careful not to cut all the way
   through the skin)
2 onions, sliced into 1cm
   (½ inch) thick rings
spray oil
1 teaspoon sumac
salt and pepper, to taste

FOR THE HOT MINT SAUCE
1 teaspoon olive oil
2 garlic cloves, crushed
½ red chilli, deseeded if you
   like, very finely chopped
½ teaspoon cumin seeds
30g (1oz) mint leaves, very finely
   chopped
2 tablespoons balsamic vinegar
2 tablespoons water
½ teaspoon sugar

1. Preheat the grill to high and arrange the lamb steaks in the middle of a large baking tray. Place the aubergines, skin side up, and sliced onions around the lamb steaks.

2. Spray the lamb, aubergines and onions lightly with oil, then place under the hot grill for 8 minutes.

3. Remove the tray from the grill, turn over the lamb steaks, aubergines and onions, sprinkle the sumac over everything and season with salt and pepper, then spray lightly with a little more oil.

4. Place the tray back under the grill for 6 minutes.

5. Meanwhile, make the hot mint sauce. Put the olive oil in a small frying pan and fry the garlic and chilli for about 30 seconds – being careful not to burn it – before adding the cumin seeds and stirring them through. Add the mint, balsamic vinegar, measured water and sugar and simmer vigorously, constantly stirring, before removing from the heat. Season with salt and pepper and set aside.

6. Remove the baking tray from under the grill and check the aubergine, to make sure that it has cooked long enough to be soft and buttery, not rubbery.

7. Place the aubergines on 2 warmed plates, then the lamb steaks on top, spoon over the onions and finally divide the hot mint sauce between the plates, spooning it over the top of the lamb and onions.

PER SERVING: Calories 477 | Fat 22g | Sat Fat 9.5g | Carbs 24g | Sugars 18g | Fibre 9.4g | Protein 40g | Salt 0.3g

SERVES 2

ONION SOUP WITH MELTED CHEDDAR

It's almost magic the amount of rich, punchy flavour that you can pull out of some simple onions. This soup has a humble list of ingredients, which mean it's easy to whip up at a moment's notice. The addition of melting Cheddar on top just adds another layer of richness. You can make this vegetarian by omitting the Worcestershire sauce and swapping the beef stock for vegetable or mushroom stock.

PREP TIME: 5 MINUTES

COOK TIME: 20 MINUTES

1 tablespoon unsalted butter

3 large onions, halved and sliced
  into half moons

4 sage leaves, finely shredded

2 garlic cloves, crushed

500ml (18fl oz) hot beef stock

1 teaspoon Worcestershire sauce

salt and pepper, to taste

30g (1oz) Cheddar cheese, grated

1. In a medium-sized saucepan, melt the butter and add the sliced onions and half the sage leaves. Fry gently, stirring occasionally, for 15 minutes until the onions are soft.

2. Stir the garlic through the onions for 30 seconds, then add the hot stock, Worcestershire sauce and some salt and pepper. Simmer for 5 minutes.

3. Blend into a smooth soup using a stick blender. (If you are freezing it, do so now, before sprinkling with the cheese.)

4. Divide the soup between 2 warmed bowls and sprinkle each with half the grated Cheddar. Grind a little black pepper over the top and finish with the rest of the shredded sage.

> **TIPS FOR STORING ONIONS**
> You can freeze sliced or chopped onions for convenient cooking. If you are preparing larger quantities, you could use the slicing attachment on a food processor or a mandoline. For chopped onions, use the blade of a food processor, but use the pulse button to avoid it turning into purée. You can freeze the onions in thick, good-quality freezer bags. Flatten them out in the bags before freezing so they stack easily. Ideal for use in soups, stews, curries and sauces.

PER SERVING: Calories 282 | Fat 12g | Sat Fat 7.3g | Carbs 31g | Sugars 23g | Fibre 8g | Protein 8.3g | Salt 1.9g

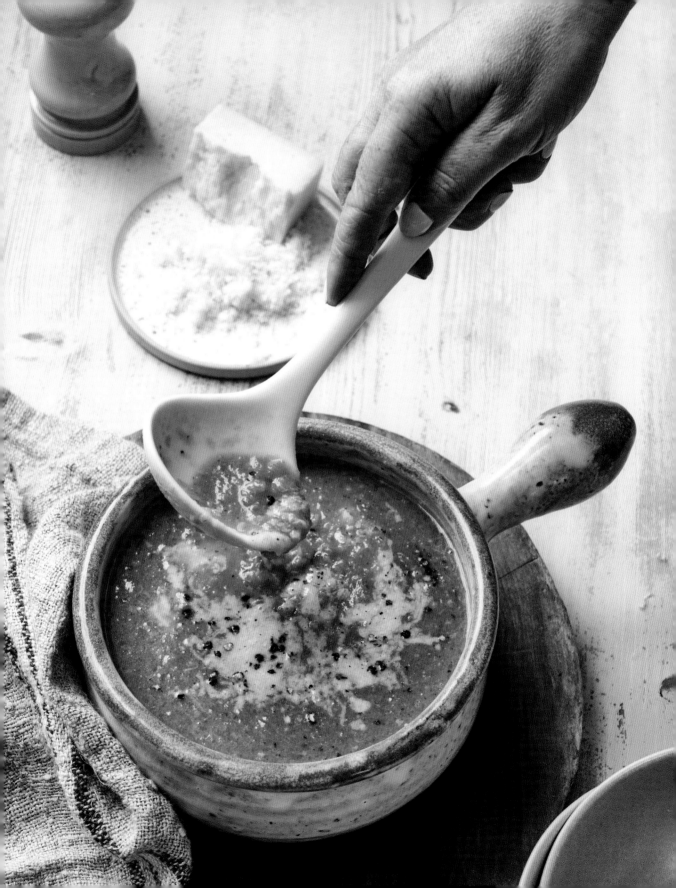

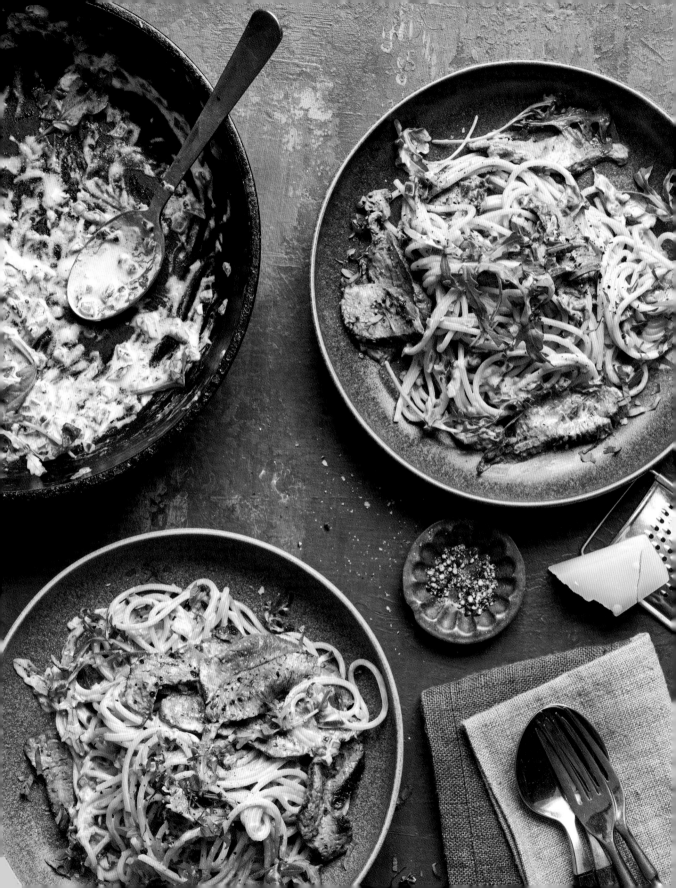

PEPPER STEAK SPAGHETTI
WITH ROCKET

**This is a lovely meal that tastes as though it should be for a special occasion,
but is easy and cost-effective enough to eat as a midweek meal.
I like my steak medium-rare in this, but if you don't like any pink,
you will need to cook the steak for a little longer.**

PREP TIME: 5 MINUTES
COOK TIME: 18 MINUTES

1 rump steak (250–300g /
    9–10½oz)
spray oil
1 large red onion, very finely
    chopped
½ teaspoon salt, plus extra for
    the steak
150g (5½oz) spaghetti
2 garlic cloves, crushed
½ teaspoon cracked black
    pepper
1 tablespoon Worcestershire
    sauce
3 tablespoons half-fat crème
    fraîche
2 large handfuls of rocket,
    roughly chopped

TO SERVE (OPTIONAL)
handful of parsley leaves, finely
    chopped
Parmesan cheese, finely grated

1. Spray the steak on each side with a little oil and season it
   with a pinch of salt.
2. Place a frying pan over a high heat and give it 30 seconds
   to heat up before adding the steak to the pan. Set a timer
   to cook this for 2½ minutes on each side for medium-rare
   (or longer if like you steak more well done) – keep the heat
   up high, the steak should be really sizzling! Remove it
   from the heat and place on a plate to rest.
3. Put the onion in the steak pan with the ½ teaspoon salt
   and fry for 2 minutes. While the onion cooks, cook the
   spaghetti in a large pan of boiling water and set a timer for
   11 minutes.
4. Add the garlic to the onion, stir it through, then take a
   ladleful of water from the pasta and add it to the frying
   pan to make sure that the garlic doesn't burn. Add the
   black pepper and Worcestershire sauce to the frying pan
   and let it gently simmer.
5. When the spaghetti has about 5 minutes of cooking time
   left, stir the crème fraîche through the sauce in the frying
   pan. Thinly slice the cooked rump steak, discarding any
   fatty bits.
6. Drain the spaghetti, add it to the frying pan, then add the
   sliced steak and the rocket and toss everything together.
7. Serve in warmed pasta bowls, with a little sprinkling of
   parsley and Parmesan, if you like.

PER SERVING: Calories 591 | Fat 16g | Sat Fat 8.3g | Carbs 64g | Sugars 9.9g | Fibre 3.9g | Protein 46g | Salt 1.9g

3 WAYS WITH COUSCOUS

Couscous is incredibly quick to cook and makes a great versatile side dish!
Serve it with proteins such as chicken, pork, beef, fish or lamb, or with
vegetarian options such as griddled halloumi, fried Portobello mushrooms
or roasted vegetables. I use wholewheat couscous for its extra fibre, as
I think it's just as nice as the white variety, but you can swap it if you like.

SERVES 4

ROSY HARISSA COUSCOUS

Harissa adds a burst of smoky, peppery flavour, so makes a great condiment
to have in the cupboard for quick meals. With crunch from the red pepper and
cooling mint, the flavours in this are versatile to accompany a wide variety
of dishes, from barbecues or grilled meat and fish, to fried halloumi, roasted
vegetables, or even a joint of meat for an alternative Sunday roast.

PREP TIME: 10 MINUTES
COOK TIME: 10 MINUTES

200g (7oz) wholewheat
   couscous
1 tablespoon harissa paste
250ml (9fl oz) boiling hot
   vegetable stock
2 red peppers, finely chopped
½ red onion, very finely chopped
150g (5½oz) cherry tomatoes,
   halved
juice of ½ lemon
large handful of mint leaves,
   finely chopped
salt and pepper, to taste

1. Place the couscous in a heatproof bowl or saucepan,
   mix in the harissa paste and pour over the boiling stock.
   Cover the bowl with a plate or a saucepan lid and leave
   for 10 minutes.

2. Meanwhile, prepare the peppers, onion and tomatoes and
   put them all into a large bowl.

3. Use a fork to fluff up the grains of couscous, then tip it
   into the bowl with the vegetables, add the lemon juice and
   mint and season with salt and pepper, then thoroughly
   mix everything together before serving.

NOTE You could add canned chickpeas, drained and rinsed,
to this to bulk it out.

PER SERVING: Calories 224 | Fat 1.9g | Sat Fat 0.3g | Carbs 40g | Sugars 8.5g | Fibre 7g | Protein 7.5g | Salt 0.8g

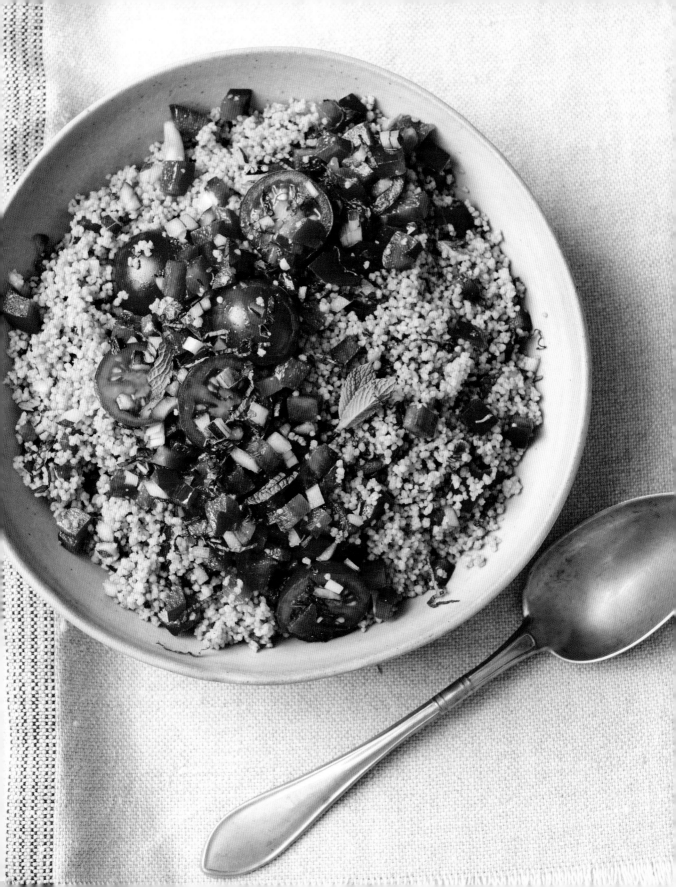

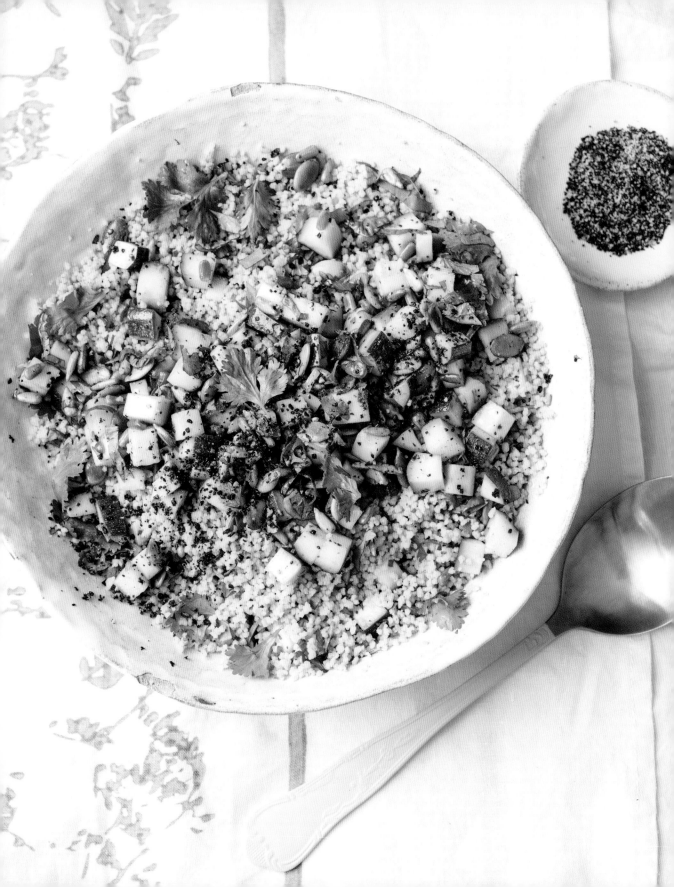

CRUNCHY COUSCOUS

Toasted seeds and little cubes of courgette add a lovely crunch to this couscous, which is also gently flavoured with sumac and lemon.

PREP TIME: 5 MINUTES
COOK TIME: 10 MINUTES

200g (7oz) wholewheat couscous
400ml (14fl oz) boiling water
2 tablespoons pumpkin seeds
2 tablespoons sunflower seeds
1 courgette, cut into small cubes
finely grated zest and juice of
    1 lemon
2 teaspoons sumac
½ teaspoon salt
¼ teaspoon pepper
large handful of coriander leaves
    and stalks, finely chopped

1. Place the couscous into a heatproof bowl or saucepan and pour over the boiled water. Cover the bowl with a plate or a saucepan lid and leave for 10 minutes.
2. Meanwhile, toast the seeds. Put them in a small frying pan and place over a medium heat. Allow them to toast (no need for oil) for about 3 minutes, stirring occasionally and keeping an eye on them to ensure they don't start to burn.
3. Once the couscous is ready, fork it through to separate the grains, then add the seeds, courgette, lemon zest and juice, sumac, salt, pepper and coriander and mix everything together. This can be eaten warm or cold.

NOTE The flavours in this will pair really well with lots of my other dishes in this book, such as Grilled Lamb & Aubergine with Hot Mint Sauce; Baked Lamb Kofta with Mint & Yogurt Sauce in Pitta; Warming Chicken & Cauliflower Curry; or Beef, Butternut & Spinach Stew (see pages 89, 125, 147, 186).

PER SERVING: Calories 275 | Fat 6.5g | Sat Fat 1g | Carbs 37g | Sugars 3.6g | Fibre 6.5g | Protein 9.9g | Salt 0.63g

CHORIZO & TOMATO COUSCOUS

A hearty couscous with crispy chorizo and herby tomatoes.

PREP TIME: 5 MINUTES
COOK TIME: 10 MINUTES

200g (7oz) wholewheat
  couscous
250ml (9fl oz) boiling hot
  chicken stock
50g (1¾oz) spicy chorizo, finely
  chopped
200g (7oz) baby tomatoes,
  halved
2 garlic cloves, crushed
2 teaspoons dried mixed herbs
salt and pepper

1. Place the couscous into a heatproof bowl or saucepan and pour over the boiling stock. Cover with a plate or saucepan lid and leave for 10 minutes. Meanwhile, cook the rest of the ingredients.

2. Place the chorizo and tomatoes in a frying pan and fry gently for 10 minutes. For the last minute of cooking, stir through the garlic and mixed herbs.

3. Once the couscous is ready, rake it through with a fork to separate the grains, then stir in the chorizo mixture and season with salt and pepper. This is delicious warm or cold.

NOTE This will pair well with Sarah's Sticky Salmon with Broccoli, Mimi's Beans or Peri-peri Chicken Cheddar Bake (see pages 70, 105, 151).

PER SERVING: Calories 242 | Fat 5.6g | Sat Fat 1.8g | Carbs 35g | Sugars 3.7g | Fibre 5g | Protein 9.9g | Salt 1.6g

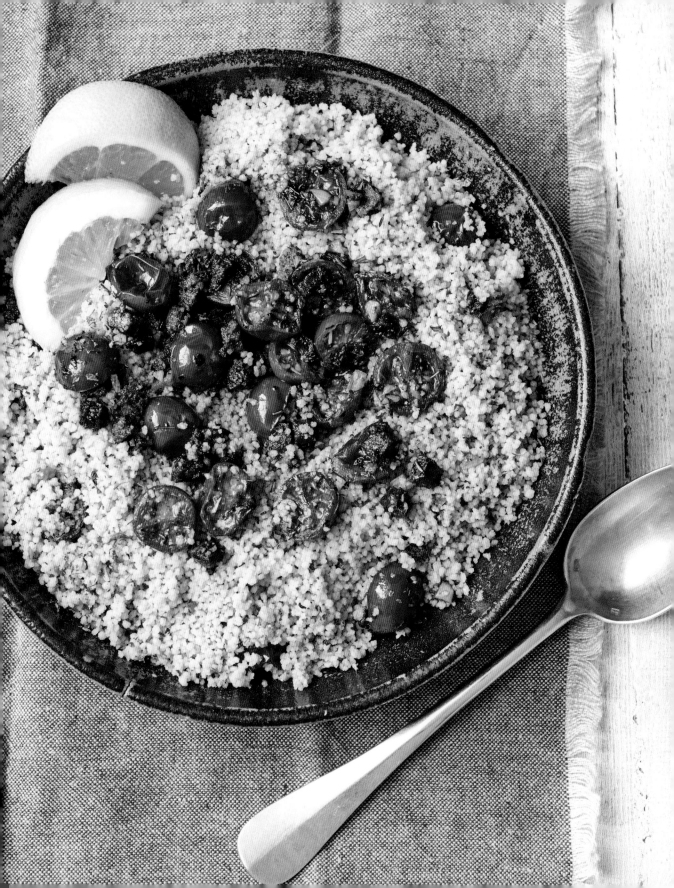

CHAPTER 4

FAMILY FAVOURITES

SERVES 4

MARLIE'S MARMITE MACARONI

Inspired by Nigella's classic spaghetti with Marmite and butter, I started making this for my youngest daughter, who loved the concept of macaroni cheese, but always found it just a bit too cheesy for her tastes. It became our go-to dinner for her and her best friend when we needed a quick tea in the evening before ballet class. Just adding in a little bit of Marmite adds great savoury flavour, while the light cheese sauce still tastes indulgent without there being an overwhelming amount of cheese to get through! We tend to serve this with some peas or broccoli on the side.

PREP TIME: 2 MINUTES
COOK TIME: 12 MINUTES

300g (10½oz) macaroni
2 teaspoons Marmite, or other
  yeast extract
50g (1¾oz) reduced-fat cream
  cheese
60g (2¼oz) Cheddar cheese,
  grated

1. Cook the macaroni in a large pan of boiling water for 12 minutes or until cooked through.
2. Drain the macaroni, reserving a little of the cooking water.
3. Spoon the Marmite and cream cheese on to the hot macaroni and stir in, adding a little bit of the reserved pasta water if you need to help it melt through a little bit.
4. Add the grated cheese and stir it through the macaroni, then serve with peas or your favourite vegetables on the side.

NOTE You can make a slightly more grown-up version of this by frying a finely chopped onion and 2 chopped bacon medallions together for about 5 minutes, then stirring them into the macaroni cheese with a couple of handfuls of roughly chopped spinach leaves.

PER SERVING: Calories 353 | Fat 8.3g | Sat Fat 4.4g | Carbs 52g | Sugars 3g |Fibre 3.8g | Protein 16g | Salt 0.84g

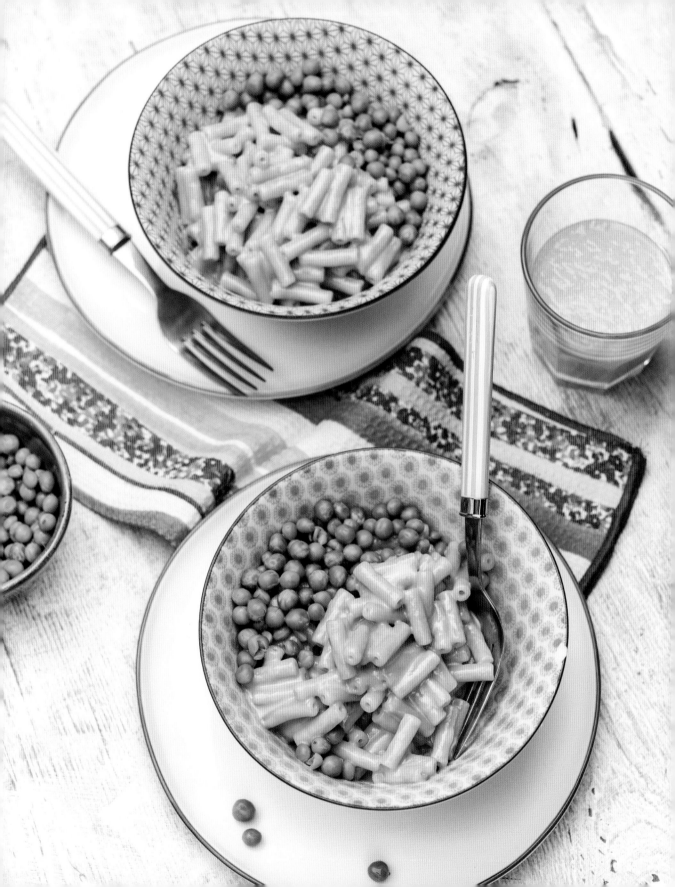

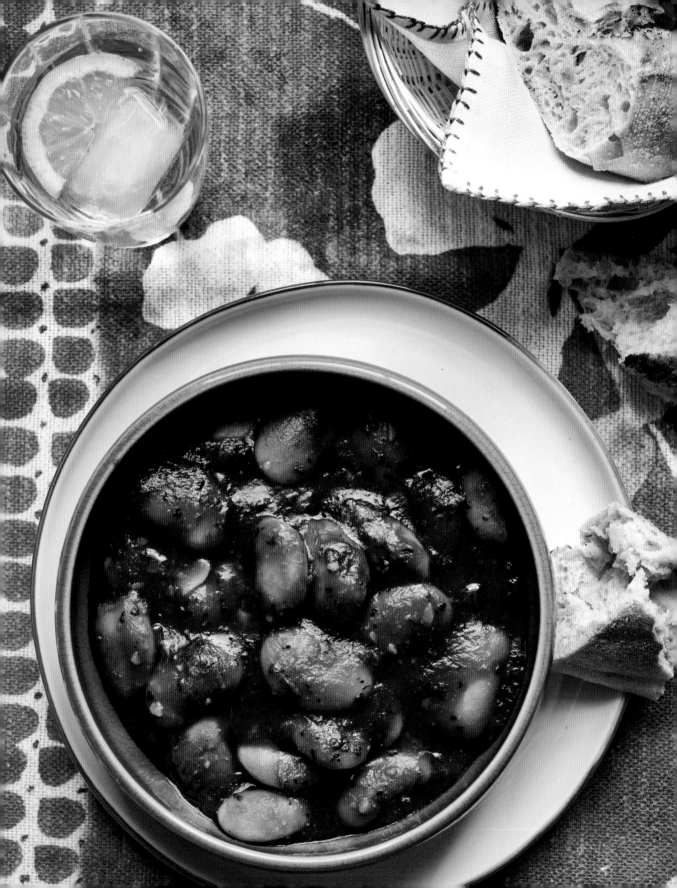

MIMI'S BEANS

These beans are my 12-year-old daughter Miette's most-requested meal! They are very simply just butter beans in a light garlic, tomato and oregano sauce, but they are really a gem of a fast meal, because they are so quick and simple to make, but also very easy to adjust into a heartier meal using what you have in the cupboards. Most often we have them on their own with fresh bread and a green vegetable such as broccoli or green beans on the side.

PREP TIME: 2 MINUTES
COOK TIME: 15 MINUTES

spray oil
4 garlic cloves, crushed
1½ teaspoons dried oregano
250g (9oz) tomato passata
100ml (3½fl oz) hot water
2 × 400g (14oz) cans of butter
    beans, drained and rinsed
salt and pepper, to taste

1. Spray a saucepan with oil and fry the garlic and oregano over a low heat for 2 minutes.
2. Add the passata and measured hot water and stir together
3. Stir through the beans and simmer over a medium heat for 12 minutes. Season and serve.

NOTE If you need these beans to be more of a substantial meal, you can stir through leftover roast chicken, or fry finely sliced chorizo or chopped bacon and add it, or simply use the beans as a side dish to accompany sausages or any other meat such as chicken, lamb or pork. My daughter loves to tear mozzarella over the top; for fussy kids, it's an easy meal that can be tailored to their tastes. You could also make a quick Cheddar or mozzarella cheese sauce to pour over and then grill it, for a bubbling cheesy bean gratin.

PER SERVING: Calories 126 | Fat 1g | Sat Fat 0.2g | Carbs 18g | Sugars 4g | Fibre 6.3g | Protein 8.3g | Salt 0.34g

HEDGEHOG CHICKEN
WITH BABY POTATOES & GREEN BEANS

Scoring chicken breasts infuses flavour into the meat, and allows it to cook quickly and evenly. You can substitute the beans with your favourite vegetables.

PREP TIME: 10 MINUTES
COOK TIME: 20 MINUTES

4 skinless chicken breasts (about 150g / 5½oz each)
3 tablespoons soy sauce
1 tablespoon honey
1 tablespoon apple cider vinegar
2 garlic cloves, crushed
spray oil
500g (1lb 2oz) baby potatoes, halved (or cut into 3 if needed, to keep a consistent size)
pinch of salt
400g (14oz) fine green beans, topped and tailed
handful of parsley leaves, very finely chopped, to serve

1. To prepare the chicken, use a sharp knife to score each chicken breast all the way across on the diagonal, cutting about three-quarters of the way through the breast, and spacing the cuts about 1cm (½ inch) apart. Then repeat, cutting diagonally across the breast in the opposite direction to create a cross-hatch pattern.
2. Mix the soy sauce, honey, apple cider vinegar and crushed garlic together in a small bowl and set aside.
3. Spray a nonstick frying pan with oil and place the chicken breasts in the pan, cross-hatch side up, handling them carefully so they don't break apart. Place over a high heat and fry for 5 minutes, then carefully flip them over and fry on the other side for 5 minutes.
4. Meanwhile, put the potatoes in a pan of simmering water, add the salt, place the lid on and simmer for 15 minutes.
5. Reduce the heat under the chicken to medium, flip the chicken breasts again so they are cross-hatch side up and pour the sauce over each breast. Cook for another 10 minutes, flipping the chicken every couple of minutes.
6. When the potatoes have been simmering for 15 minutes, add the green beans to the pan (make sure there is enough water so they are submerged) and cook for a final 5 minutes.
7. Check that the chicken breasts are fully cooked through with no pink remaining (or use a meat thermometer to be sure that they are fully cooked, see page 109). Drain the potatoes and beans and divide between 4 warmed plates, then add a chicken breast to each plate and scatter with the parsley.

PER SERVING: Calories 268 | Fat 2.5g | Sat Fat 0.6g | Carbs 28g | Sugars 10g | Fibre 5.7g | Protein 30g | Salt 2.1g

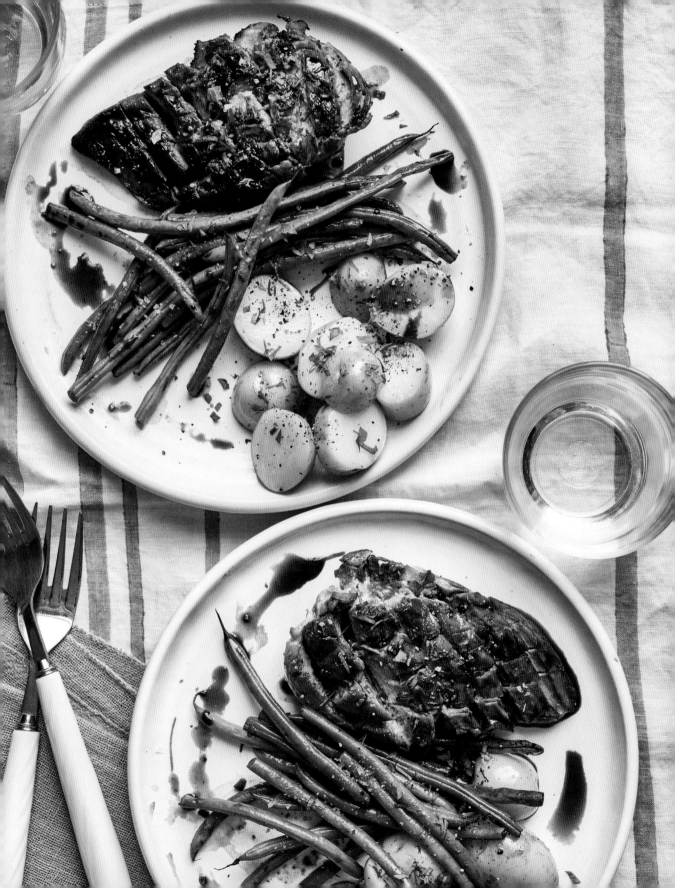

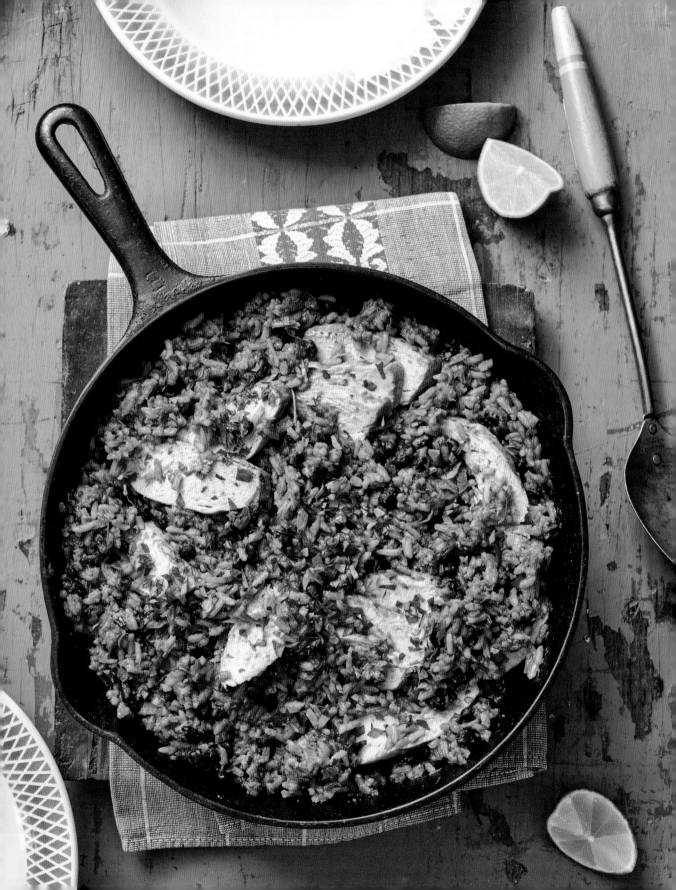

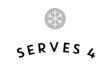

CHICKEN SALSA RICE

A lovely, easy one-pot rice dish that makes an easy family-friendly meal. As I make this for my chilli-averse children, I don't add any spice while I'm cooking it, but scatter on some jalapeños or add a squeeze of chilli sauce to my portion at the table.

PREP TIME: 5 MINUTES
COOK TIME: 25 MINUTES

spray oil
3 spring onions, sliced
2 skinless chicken breasts
400ml (14fl oz) hot chicken
 stock
200g (7oz) white long grain rice
400g (14oz) can of black beans,
 drained and rinsed
400g (14oz) can of chopped
 tomatoes
100g (3½oz) frozen sweetcorn
1 teaspoon garlic granules
1 teaspoon onion granules
1 teaspoon ground cumin
1 teaspoon dried oregano
½ teaspoon salt

TO SERVE
lime wedges
handful of parsley leaves,
 finely chopped

1. Spray a sauté pan (for which you have a lid) with oil and fry the spring onions and whole chicken breasts for 3 minutes, turning the breasts a couple of times to lightly brown each side.
2. Pour the hot stock into the pan, bring to a simmer and add all the other ingredients.
3. Simmer for 20 minutes, turning the chicken breasts over after 10 minutes.
4. After 20 minutes check the chicken is cooked through (see tip below), then remove from the heat, place a lid on and leave to rest for 2 minutes.
5. Remove the chicken breasts and finely slice them, then stir back into the rice. Serve with lime wedges and parsley.

TIPS ON PREPARING CHICKEN
It's really important to check that chicken is properly cooked. Chicken breasts can vary hugely in size, and cooking time can also depend on whether the chicken is at room temperature or has just come out of the refrigerator. Ideally take your chicken breasts out of the refrigerator up to 30 minutes before cooking them. You can visually check that chicken is cooked through by making sure there is no pink flesh, but the best way is to check it with a meat thermometer. Insert the thermometer into the thickest part of the breast: the internal temperature should be at least 74°C (165°F).

PER SERVING: Calories 401 | Fat 3.7g | Sat Fat 0.6g | Carbs 58g | Sugars 9.9g | Fibre 7.9g | Protein 29g | Salt 2.6g

PESTO CHICKEN MACARONI

WITH BROCCOLI

Macaroni is one of my daughters' favourite pasta shapes – maybe because it's bite-sized and easy to eat – so we use it for a lot more than macaroni cheese. The bonus for a quick meal is that it cooks faster than some other pastas, so I use it for many family meals.

PREP TIME: 5 MINUTES
COOK TIME: 25 MINUTES

6 skinless chicken thigh fillets,
    excess fat trimmed away
250g (9oz) baby tomatoes
1 onion, finely chopped
150ml (¼ pint) hot chicken
    stock
2 tablespoons green pesto
    (see note)
300g (10½oz) macaroni
½ head of broccoli, broken into
    florets
salt and pepper, to taste

TO SERVE
Parmesan cheese, finely grated
lemon wedges

1. Preheat the oven to 220°C/200°C fan (425°F), Gas Mark 7.
2. Put the chicken in a medium-large ovenproof serving dish that will fit all the ingredients and the cooked macaroni. Add the tomatoes, onion, hot stock and pesto and stir everything together, then season with salt and pepper.
3. Place in the oven for 25 minutes.
4. After the chicken has been cooking for 10 minutes, fill a large saucepan with plenty of boiling water (you need enough to cook the macaroni and the broccoli).
5. Simmer the macaroni for 7 minutes, then add the broccoli and simmer for a further 5 minutes. Drain.
6. Remove the dish from the oven and check the chicken is cooked through (see tip on page 109). Finely slice the chicken with a sharp knife, then stir it back into the dish along with with the macaroni and broccoli.
7. Sprinkle with Parmesan and serve with lemon wedges on the side.

NOTE You can make this with any of my Pesto variations (see pages 128–133), for a different-tasting meal every time. You can add as many extra quick-cook vegetables as you like to this dish depending on everyone's favourites; try peas, green beans, asparagus spears, sugarsnap peas or mangetout.

PER SERVING: Calories 539 | Fat 16g | Sat Fat 3.7g | Carbs 59g | Sugars 8.4g | Fibre 7.9g | Protein 34g | Salt 1.3g

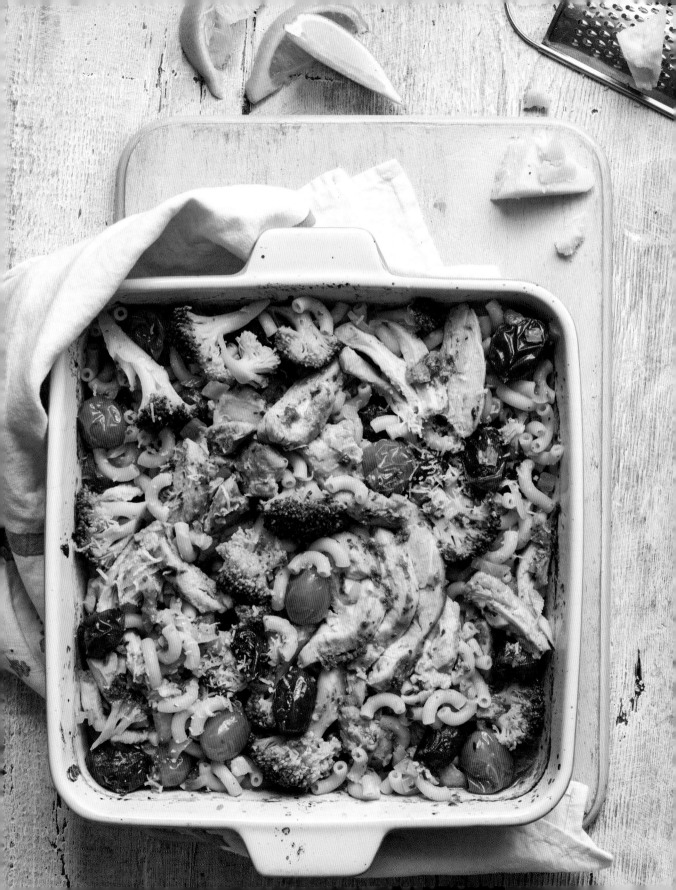

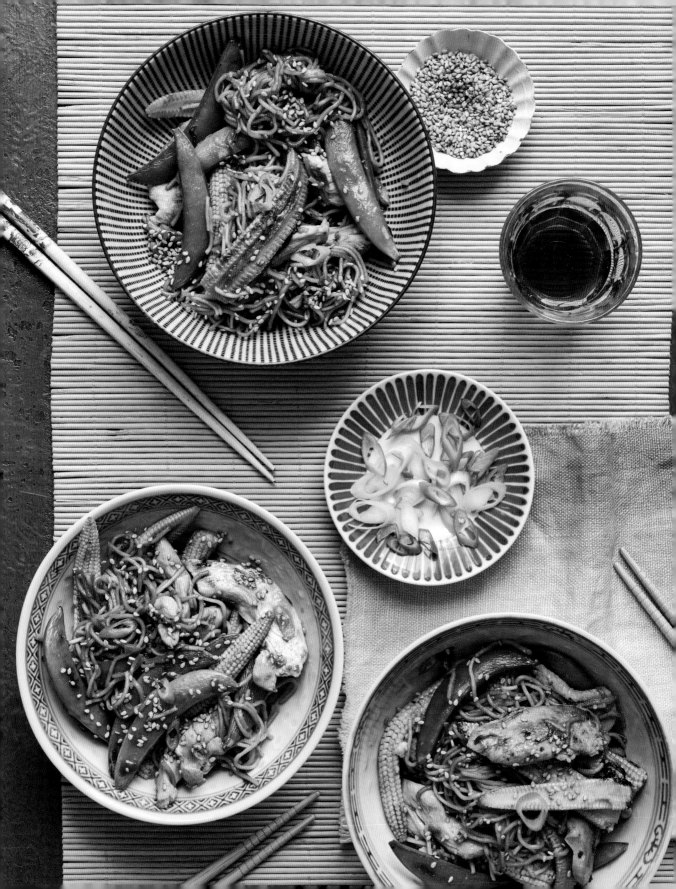

SIMPLE BABY CORN & CHICKEN STIR-FRY

WITH HONEY SOY DRESSING

My girls don't like overpowering flavours in stir-fries, so this is the simple recipe that I make for us to eat, moan-free, as a family. It's tasty enough for the grown-ups to enjoy it, but simple enough for fussy eaters, with no hidden surprises.

PREP TIME: 5 MINUTES
COOK TIME: 10 MINUTES

1 teaspoon toasted sesame oil
2 skinless chicken breasts, finely sliced
3 nests of fine egg noodles
175g (6oz) baby sweetcorn, halved lengthways
2 spring onions, finely sliced
160g (5¾oz) sugarsnap peas
sesame seeds, to serve

FOR THE DRESSING
2 tablespoons light soy sauce
1 tablespoon honey
1 tablespoon Shaoxing rice wine

1. Make up the dressing in a small bowl by mixing all the ingredients.
2. Heat a wok or sauté pan over a high heat, add the oil and stir-fry the chicken for 5 minutes until cooked through.
3. Meanwhile, break the noodle nests in half and submerge them in a pan of boiling water to simmer for 4 minutes (or cook according to the packet instructions, if they differ).
4. While the noodles are cooking, add the baby sweetcorn to the wok with the spring onions and sugarsnap peas and stir-fry over a medium heat.
5. Drain the noodles and add them to the wok, then tip in the dressing, reduce the heat to low and stir everything together until well mixed and the noodles are lightly coated in the sauce.
6. Serve with a sprinkling of sesame seeds on top.

NOTE Baby sweetcorn is always popular in my house, as are crunchy sugarsnap peas, but you can tailor the vegetables in this to whatever your kids will happily eat. Sometimes I add raw carrot cut into matchsticks at the end, or swap out the sugarsnaps for fine green beans or broccoli (we eat our broccoli crunchy, but if you like it softer, then simmer it for a few minutes and stir it in at the end).

PER SERVING: Calories 280 | Fat 3.2g | Sat Fat 0.9g | Carbs 36g | Sugars 9.8g | Fibre 3.3g | Protein 25g | Salt 2.2g

CHICKEN SAUSAGES WITH CREAMY LENTILS

Chicken sausages are a great family-friendly dish for two reasons: they tend to be leaner than pork sausages, and they have a mild flavour that is great for kids and also won't overpower a dish. I blend all of the vegetables in this so that they aren't discernible among the lentil and sausages, for an easy-to-eat family favourite. I usually serve this for the kids in mini casserole dishes with some crusty French bread.

PREP TIME: 5 MINUTES

COOK TIME: 18 MINUTES

1 onion, quartered

1 leek, trimmed (see page 43) and outer leaves removed, cut into 3

1 celery stick, cut into 3

1 carrot, cut into 3

leaves from 1 rosemary sprig

2 garlic cloves

spray oil

8 chicken chipolatas, each sliced into 6

250ml (9fl oz) hot chicken stock

2 × 400g (14oz) cans of green lentils, drained and rinsed

4 tablespoons single cream

salt and pepper, to taste

1. Use a food processor to pulse-chop the onion, leek, celery, carrot, rosemary and garlic until all are very finely chopped.

2. Spray a sauté pan with oil and fry the sausage pieces for 3 minutes to give them some colour, then add all the finely chopped vegetables with some salt and pepper and fry these for 10 minutes, stirring frequently.

3. Pour the hot stock into the pan, add the lentils and simmer gently for 5 minutes.

4. Stir the cream through the lentils and serve.

NOTE If you want to substitute the chicken sausages for vegetarian sausages, cook them separately according to the packet instructions, then slice and add to the creamy lentils, and use vegetable stock in place of chicken stock to keep the whole meal vegetarian.

PER SERVING: Calories 287 | Fat 12g | Sat Fat 4.1g | Carbs 20g | Sugars 3.6g | Fibre 8.2g | Protein 21g | Salt 2.1g

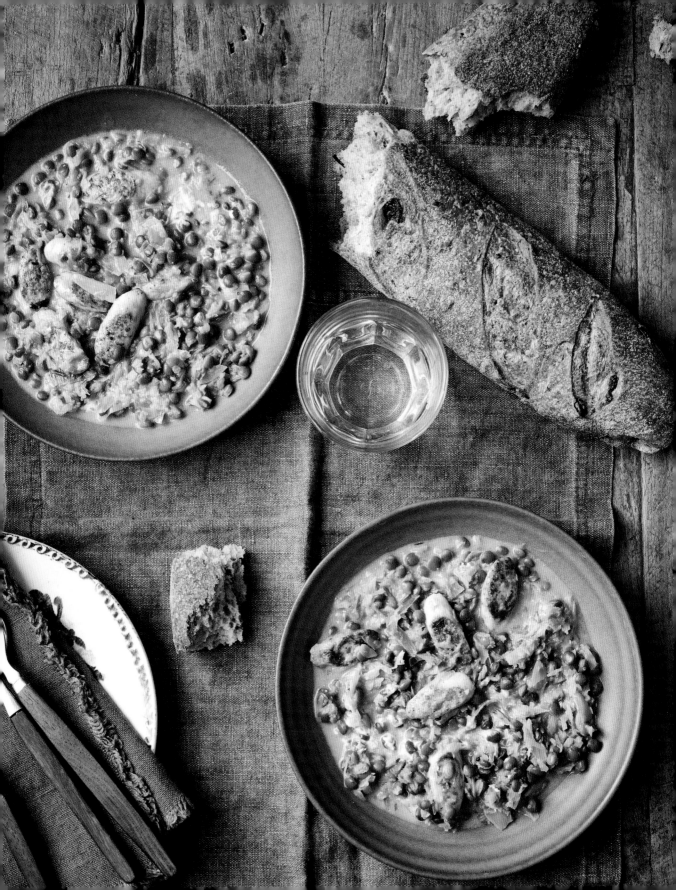

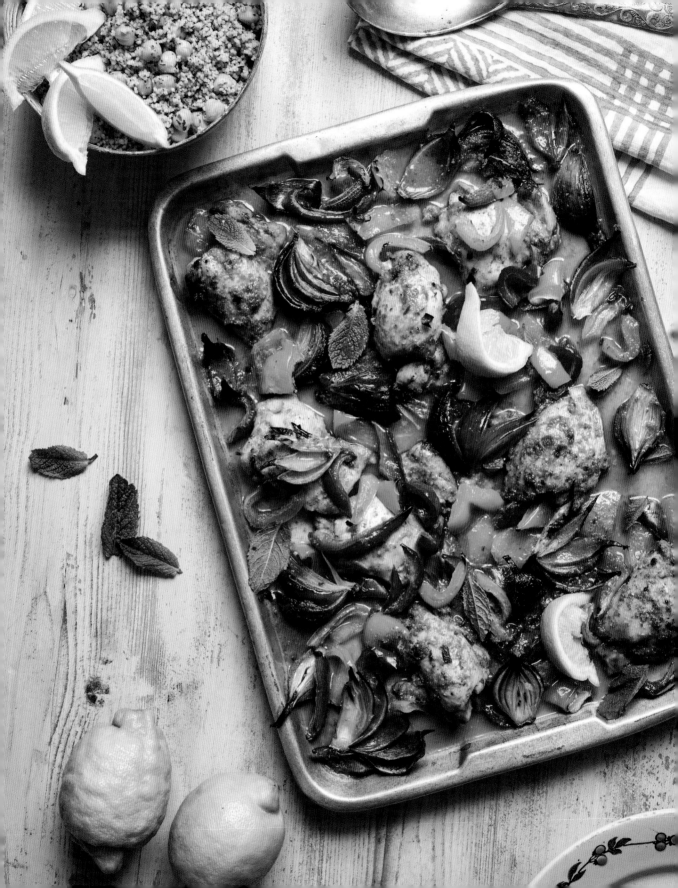

MOROCCAN-STYLE CHICKEN THIGHS

WITH MINTED CHICKPEA COUSCOUS

Zesty, sweet and spicy chicken thighs and roasted vegetables are complemented by minty couscous with a hint of cinnamon.

PREP TIME: 10 MINUTES

COOK TIME: 20 MINUTES

8 skinless chicken thigh fillets, excess fat trimmed away

2 red onions, cut into wedges

1 red pepper, finely sliced

1 yellow pepper, finely sliced

spray oil

lemon wedges, to serve

FOR THE SAUCE

2 tablespoons pure maple syrup

finely grated zest and juice of 1 orange

finely grated zest and juice of 1 lemon

1 tablespoon harissa paste

1 teaspoon ground cumin

1 teaspoon garlic granules

pinch of salt

FOR THE COUSCOUS

400g (14oz) can of chickpeas, drained and rinsed

2 tablespoons dried mint

¼ teaspoon ground cinnamon

200g (7oz) wholewheat couscous

300ml (½ pint) boiling chicken stock

mint leaves, to serve (optional)

1. Preheat the oven to 210°C/190°C fan (410°F), Gas Mark 6½.

2. Mix the sauce ingredients together in a bowl.

3. Place the chicken thigh fillets, red onion wedges and peppers into a baking tray or roasting tin and spoon the sauce over everything. Spritz with spray oil and put into the oven for 20 minutes.

4. After the chicken has cooked for 10 minutes, mix the chickpeas, dried mint and cinnamon into the dry couscous in a saucepan or heatproof bowl, then pour over the boiling stock, cover and leave for 10 minutes.

5. Remove the chicken from the oven and check it is cooked through (see page 109).

6. Fluff up the couscous with a fork and serve into 4 warmed bowls. Spoon the chicken, veg and juices over the couscous. Serve with lemon wedges and mint leaves scattered over, if you like.

> **TIPS ON STORING LEMONS**
>
> If you have leftover lemon wedges, or whole lemons that are soon going to go out of date, cut any whole lemons into wedges, pop into an airtight freezer-safe container or freezer bag and freeze until you need them. You can also do this with limes. This saves waste and means you always have lemon and lime wedges on hand.

PER SERVING: Calories 577 | Fat 15g | Sat Fat 3.8g | Carbs 63g | Sugars 20g | Fibre 11g | Protein 41g | Salt 2.7g

SERVES 4

SAUSAGE BALLS WITH ORZO & BEANS

Simple sausage meatballs always go down a treat with my children, while adding easy-to-eat orzo and haricot beans with simple flavours turn them into a great, balanced meal.

PREP TIME: 10 MINUTES
COOK TIME: 20 MINUTES

500g (1lb 2oz) lean minced pork
(5 per cent fat)
1 tablespoon Italian-style mixed
dried herbs
1 carrot, grated
1 teaspoon baking powder
¼ teaspoon salt
spray oil
200g (7oz) orzo pasta
400g (14oz) can of haricot beans,
drained and rinsed
600ml (20fl oz) hot chicken
stock
2 celery sticks, finely chopped
1 onion, finely chopped
2 garlic cloves, crushed
2 tablespoons tomato ketchup
1 teaspoon dried thyme
½ teaspoon fennel seeds
2 large handfuls of kale leaves,
coarse stalks removed,
roughly chopped

1. To make the meatballs, mix the pork, dried herbs, carrot, baking powder and ¼ teaspoon salt in a bowl. Use your hands to shape the mixture into walnut-sized balls (3cm/1¼ inches in diameter – no need for perfection here, just a roughly round shape is fine!). I make about 22 meatballs with this mixture. As you make them, place them directly into a large sauté or frying pan, off the heat, which has been sprayed with a little oil.

2. Put the orzo and haricot beans into a saucepan, pour over the hot stock and simmer for 15 minutes, stirring occasionally to prevent the orzo sticking to the bottom of the pan.

3. Place the sauté pan containing the sausage balls over a high heat and start to fry, add the celery, onion and garlic, reduce the heat to medium and cook, stirring occasionally.

4. After the orzo has been cooking for 15 minutes, tip the entire contents of the pan into the sauté pan and carefully mix everything together (try not to break up the meatballs).

5. Add the ketchup, thyme, fennel seeds and kale to the pan and stir together. Simmer gently for another 5 minutes before serving.

NOTE If you don't eat pork, you could substitute minced chicken or turkey.

PER SERVING: Calories 473 | Fat 8.7g | Sat Fat 2.6g | Carbs 55g | Sugars 8.1g | Fibre 6.2g | Protein 40g | Salt 3.6g

118 | FAMILY FAVOURITES

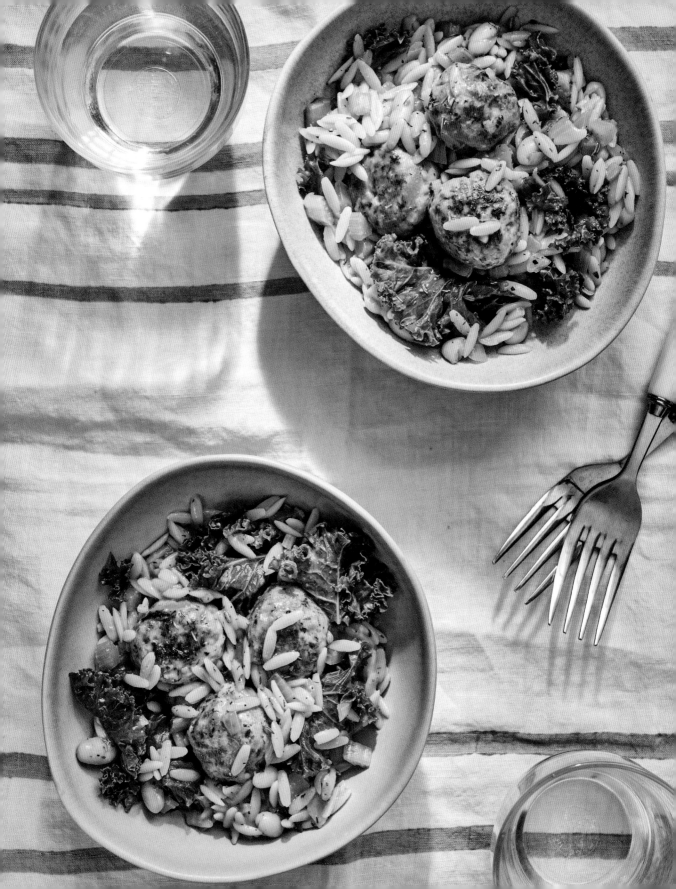

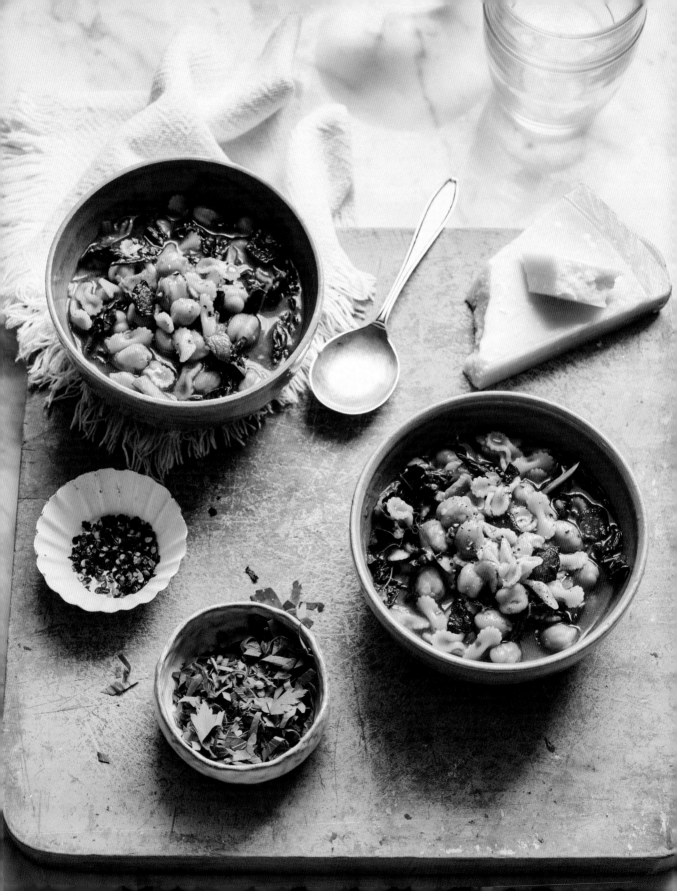

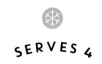

PASTA E CECI

This is my take on the popular hearty Italian soup of pasta and chickpeas, which I first tried in Rome. This is a great meal for kids as it has subtle flavours and small, easy-to-manage pasta shapes. You can also make this vegetarian by omitting the bacon.

PREP TIME: 5 MINUTES
COOK TIME: 20 MINUTES

spray oil
4 smoked bacon medallions, finely chopped
1 red onion, finely chopped
2 garlic cloves, crushed
1 tablespoon rosemary leaves, finely chopped
1 litre (1¾ pints) hot white wine stock (see note)
2 × 400g (14oz) cans of chickpeas, drained and rinsed
150g (5½oz) soup pasta such as ditalini, mini shells or orzo
1 tablespoon tomato purée
2 handfuls of kale leaves, coarse stalks removed, roughly chopped
pepper, to taste

TO SERVE
Parmesan, or Parmesan-style vegetarian cheese, finely grated
handful of parsley leaves, finely chopped
pinch of chilli flakes (optional)

1. Spray a large saucepan with oil and stir-fry the bacon, onion, garlic and rosemary for 3 minutes.
2. Pour in the hot stock, add the chickpeas and pasta, stir in the tomato purée, then simmer for 10 minutes, stirring every now and again to make sure the pasta doesn't stick to the bottom of the pan.
3. Add the kale, season with pepper and simmer for a further 5 minutes. By this time the pasta should be cooked (just taste a piece to check). Depending on what pasta you use, you may need to add a little extra stock or boiling water at this stage.
4. Serve in bowls scattered with Parmesan, parsley and chilli flakes, if you like.

NOTE I have suggested white wine stock, which is available in some supermarkets, but if you can't get hold of any then chicken or vegetable stock will work just fine. In some versions of this recipe, a ladleful of cooked chickpeas and stock is removed, blended, then stirred back in to make a creamier, thicker-textured soup. I haven't added that step to keep this version quick, but you might prefer it that way. You can add extra veg of your choice, such as celery fried at the same time as the onions, or finely chopped carrots. You could also replace the bacon with a couple of anchovies.

PER SERVING: Calories 389 | Fat 6.4g | Sat Fat 0.8g | Carbs 55g | Sugars 8g | Fibre 8.5g | Protein 23g | Salt 2.9g

ALL-ABOUT-THE-GRAVY SAUSAGE & MASH

Sausage, mash and onion gravy has always been one of my favourites. The gravy here is simple to cook and tastes great: packed with soft fried onions and sausage pieces, it makes a really satisfying meal. The secret to quick mash is cutting the potatoes into small chunks before boiling them. Serve with kale, peas, or any other quick-cooking vegetables of your choice.

PREP TIME: 10 MINUTES

COOK TIME: 20 MINUTES

800g (1lb 12oz) white potatoes, cut into small chunks

spray oil

8 reduced-fat pork sausages, each sliced into 6

2 onions, halved and finely sliced into half moons

300g (10½ oz) chestnut mushrooms, halved or quartered if large

500ml (18fl oz) beef stock

2 tablespoons tomato purée

1 tablespoon brown sauce, such as HP

1 teaspoon dried sage

1 tablespoon cornflour

3 tablespoons cold water

50ml (1¾fl oz) semi-skimmed milk

salt and pepper, to taste

1. Put the potato chunks into a large pan of boiling water and simmer for 15–20 minutes until tender.
2. Spray a sauté pan with oil and fry the sausage pieces, onions and mushrooms, stirring occasionally, for 10 minutes.
3. While the sausages are frying, make up the gravy. Pour the beef stock into a jug, add the tomato purée, brown sauce and sage and mix together. Dissolve the cornflour in the cold water in a small bowl and stir to ensure there are no lumps, then pour this into the jug.
4. Pour the gravy into the pan with the sausages and allow to simmer gently for 5 minutes while the potatoes finish cooking, stirring occasionally. Taste the gravy and add salt and pepper if needed.
5. Drain the potatoes, allow them to steam off for a couple of minutes, then mash them with the milk and salt and pepper until smooth and lump-free.
6. Serve the mashed potatoes and sausage gravy with your vegetables of choice.

NOTE You can jazz up the mashed potato by stirring through a couple of teaspoons of wholegrain mustard or horseradish sauce, or mix through some grated cheese. You could also add chopped herbs such as parsley or chives.

PER SERVING: Calories 354 | Fat 6.1g | Sat Fat 2g | Carbs 53g | Sugars 11g | Fibre 6.9g | Protein 18g | Salt 2.9g

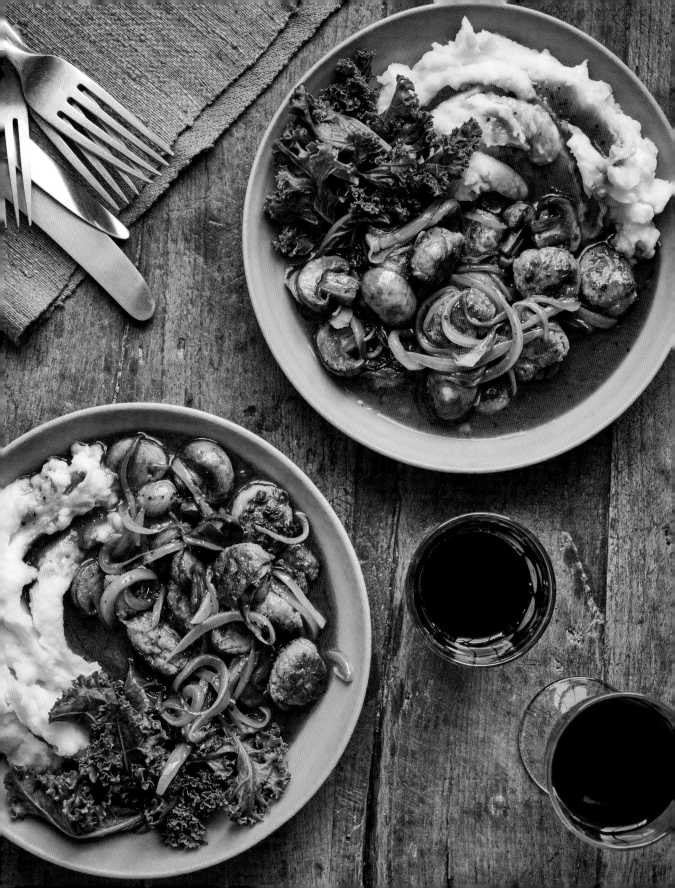

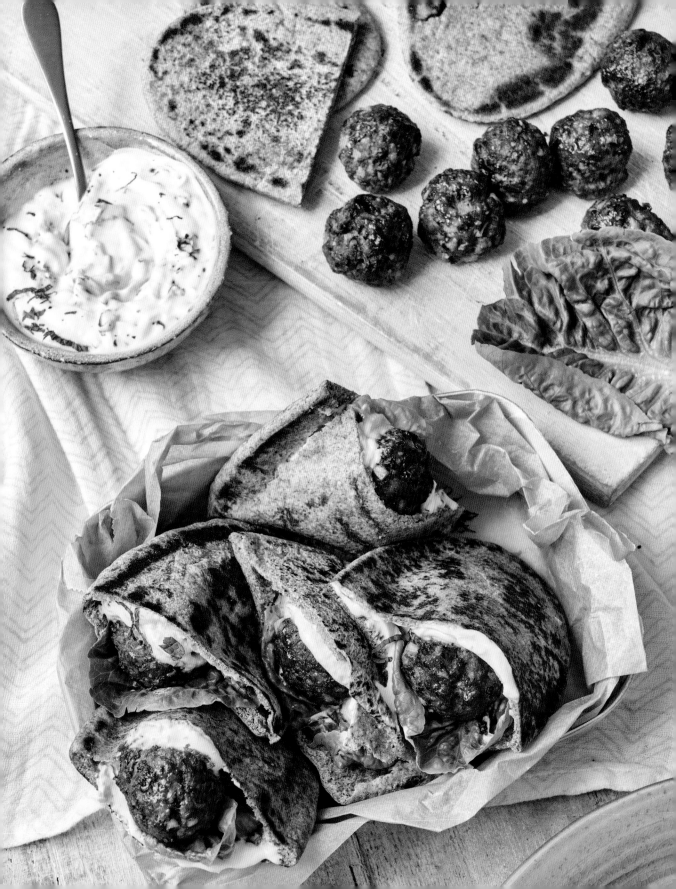

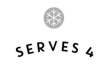

BAKED LAMB KOFTA
WITH MINT & YOGURT SAUCE IN PITTA

Lamb kofta are always an easy win with my kids. Shaping the kofta into balls and baking them is quicker than cooking on skewers, when they often fall apart. I sometimes serve them with salad and homemade fries, or simply serve with rice and vegetables. The koftas also go well with all my Couscous recipes (see pages 94–99) and hummus.

PREP TIME: 10 MINUTES
COOK TIME: 15 MINUTES

500g (1lb 2oz) lean minced lamb
    (10 per cent fat)
1 onion, grated
2 garlic cloves, crushed
2 teaspoons ground cumin
1 teaspoon ground coriander
½ teaspoon ground allspice
½ teaspoon salt
½ teaspoon pepper
large handful of parsley leaves,
    finely chopped
4 wholemeal pitta breads
salad leaves of your choice,
    to serve (optional)

FOR THE MINT & YOGURT SAUCE
250g (9oz) fat-free Greek yogurt
small handful of mint leaves,
    finely chopped
juice of ½ lemon
pinch of salt

1. Preheat the oven to 240°C/220°C fan (475°F), Gas Mark 9.
2. In a large bowl, mix together the lamb, onion, garlic, cumin, coriander, allspice, salt, pepper and parsley until thoroughly combined.
3. Using your hands, shape the mixture into balls about 3cm (1¼ inches) in diameter (this will make 14–16 balls) and place on a baking tray (you can use a roasting tin with a rack, to allow the fat to drain away).
4. Pop in the oven and roast for 15 minutes, by which time they should be browning and caramelizing on the outside, but still tender in the middle.
5. Meanwhile, mix all the ingredients for the mint and yogurt sauce together in a bowl.
6. Toast the pitta breads (I use the toaster, but you could pop them briefly into the oven too).
7. Slice open the pittas, add a couple of teaspoons of the sauce and spread inside, then pop 2–3 koftas into each, along with any salad items of choice, then serve. I also put out the sauce and remaining koftas on the table so everyone can help themselves, or you can freeze leftover koftas.

NOTE For a cheeky little addition, stuff the kofta with some feta cheese. Simply cut 50g (1¾oz) feta into 1cm (½ inch) cubes and form the kofta into balls, each with a cube of feta at its centre.

PER SERVING: Calories 480 | Fat 14g | Sat Fat 6g | Carbs 42g | Sugars 7.2g | Fibre 5.9g | Protein 4.3g | Salt 2g

BEEF & GNOCCHI RAGU

An easy, comfort food one-pot with a simple Bolognese-style sauce with tender gnocchi. Use a food processor or mini chopper to make the easy sauce and save on chopping. You don't have to add the final step of stirring in cheese, you can always serve up grated cheese on the side for people to add if they want.

PREP TIME: 5 MINUTES
COOK TIME: 20 MINUTES

400g (14oz) can of chopped
    tomatoes
3 garlic cloves
1 tablespoon Italian-style mixed
    dried herbs
1 carrot, roughly chopped into
    2cm (¾ inch) pieces (no need
    to peel)
spray oil
500g (1lb 2oz) lean minced beef
    (5 per cent fat)
1 onion, finely chopped
2 celery sticks, finely chopped
2 tablespoons tomato purée
1 teaspoon dried rosemary
250ml (9fl oz) hot red wine
    stock (see note on page 121),
    or beef stock
500g (1lb 2oz) fresh gnocchi
60g (2¼oz) Cheddar cheese,
    grated
salt and pepper, to taste
handful of basil leaves or parsley
    leaves, finely chopped, to serve

1. In a food processor or mini chopper, make up the sauce by blending together the chopped tomatoes, garlic, dried herbs and carrot.

2. Spray a large sauté pan or shallow flameproof casserole dish with oil and stir-fry the beef, onion and celery for 5 minutes, breaking apart any clumps of beef.

3. Add the tomato sauce, tomato purée, rosemary and stock, stir everything together and simmer for 5 minutes.

4. Now add the gnocchi and simmer for another 10 minutes, stirring occasionally.

5. Stir in the Cheddar, season with salt and pepper and serve with the herbs on top.

NOTE If you prefer, you can sprinkle the cheese on the top of the dish and grill it for a bubbling, cheesy top. Mozzarella and Parmesan will also work well here, instead of (or as well as) Cheddar.

PER SERVING: Calories 306 | Fat 12g | Sat Fat 6g | Carbs 12g | Sugars 10g | Fibre 3.8g | Protein 35g | Salt 1.3g

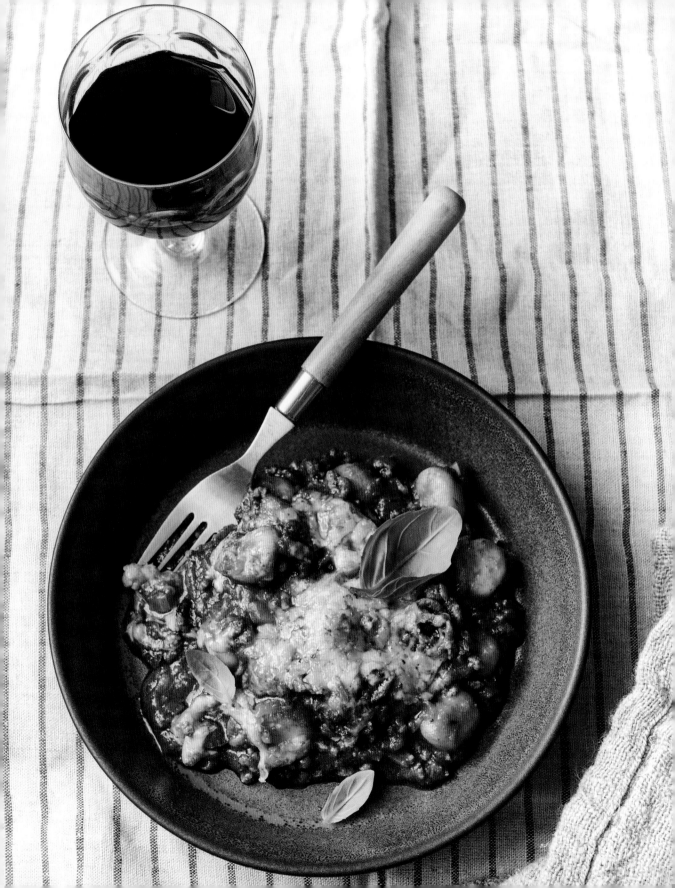

3 WAYS WITH PESTO

Pesto is a fabulous flavour enhancer and can be used for meals in a variety of ways. These three different pestos can offer a huge variety of options:

+ Mixed through pasta
+ Spread on salmon fillets or chicken breasts
+ Mixed through roasted vegetables
+ Spread in pitta breads, on crackers, or in a cheese toastie
+ Swirled through soup
+ Added to mini frittatas
+ Mixed into hummus
+ Stirred through risotto
+ With fried eggs (see page 24), or stirred through scrambled egg
+ Added to salad dressing

SERVES 4

BLUSHING RED PEPPER PESTO

Classic basil and Parmesan pesto flavours with the added sweetness of roasted red pepper and a hint of red chilli. I use pumpkin seeds in this, which are much cheaper than pine nuts and work really well here.

PREP TIME: 5 MINUTES
COOK TIME: NONE

1 roasted red pepper in brine,
    from a jar, drained
1 garlic clove, peeled
handful of basil leaves
2 tablespoons pumpkin seeds
30g (1oz) Parmesan cheese,
    roughly cut up
1 red chilli, deseeded
½ teaspoon salt

1. Put all the ingredients into a mini chopper or small food processor bowl and blend until combined into a smooth pesto.

NOTE Roasted red peppers in brine packed into jars are a magic ingredient that are ready to go! Roasting your own peppers creates great flavour, but can be a little labour intensive. I use red peppers from a jar in curries, sauces, pasta dishes, frittatas, pitta breads and salads; they are incredibly versatile.

PER SERVING: Calories 91 | Fat 5.1g | Sat Fat 1.9g | Carbs 4.8g | Sugars 3.8g | Fibre 1.1g | Protein 5.8g | Salt 0.74g

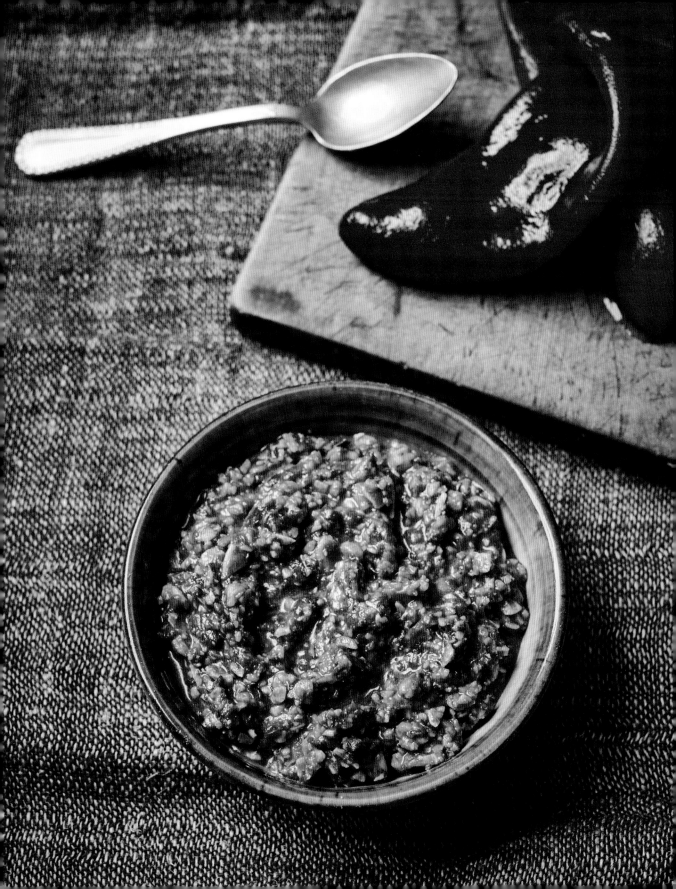

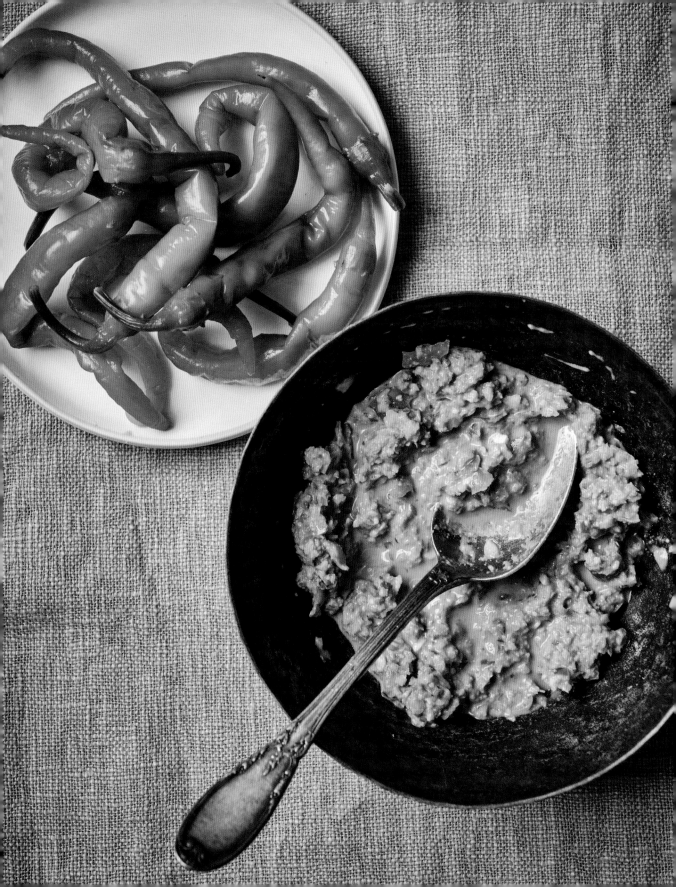

PUNCHY PICKLED CHILLI & WALNUT PESTO

This one really is a flavour explosion. I tend to use it on vegetables, meat and grains such as bulgur wheat, rather than mixed through pasta.

PREP TIME: 5 MINUTES
COOK TIME: NONE

3 pickled chillies, stalks removed
finely grated zest and juice of
    1 lemon
20g (¾oz) walnuts
1 garlic clove
10g (¼oz) nutritional yeast
1 tablespoon red wine vinegar
1 teaspoon salt
½ teaspoon ground turmeric

1. Put all the ingredients into a mini chopper or small food processor bowl and blend until combined into a smooth pesto.

NOTE You will find pickled chillies in jars in the supermarket in the same place as the olives and roasted peppers in brine. They are hot and sour and make a great flavour booster.

PER SERVING: Calories 60 | Fat 3.7g | Sat Fat 0.4g | Carbs 1.8g | Sugars 1.6g | Fibre 1.2g | Protein 3g | Salt 1.4g

VEGAN KALE & CASHEW PESTO

An extra-healthy pesto, this is packed with flavour and makes a great flavour-base for a vegan-friendly meal. Nutritional yeast takes the place of Parmesan in this, as it has a cheesy, nutty flavour.

PREP TIME: 5 MINUTES
COOK TIME: NONE

4 handfuls of kale leaves, coarse
    stalks removed, chopped
    (total weight about 55g / 2oz)
1 garlic clove
10g (¼oz) nutritional yeast
juice of 1 lemon
40g (1½oz) cashew nuts
1 cherry tomato
½ teaspoon olive oil
1 teaspoon salt
¼ teaspoon cracked black pepper

1. Put all the ingredients into a mini chopper or small food processor bowl and blend until combined into a smooth pesto.

NOTE Nutritional yeast is a great ingredient to add cheesy, savoury flavour to vegan dishes. With the huge surge in popularity of veganism, it has become much more readily available and you should find it easy to get hold of in many supermarkets and health food shops. You can also add it to pasta dishes in place of Parmesan, sprinkle it over soup for extra flavour, or mix it into vegan stews or risottos.

PER SERVING: Calories 82 | Fat 5.7g | Sat Fat 1.1g | Carbs 2.6g | Sugars 1.2g | Fibre 1.6g | Protein 4g | Salt 0.64g

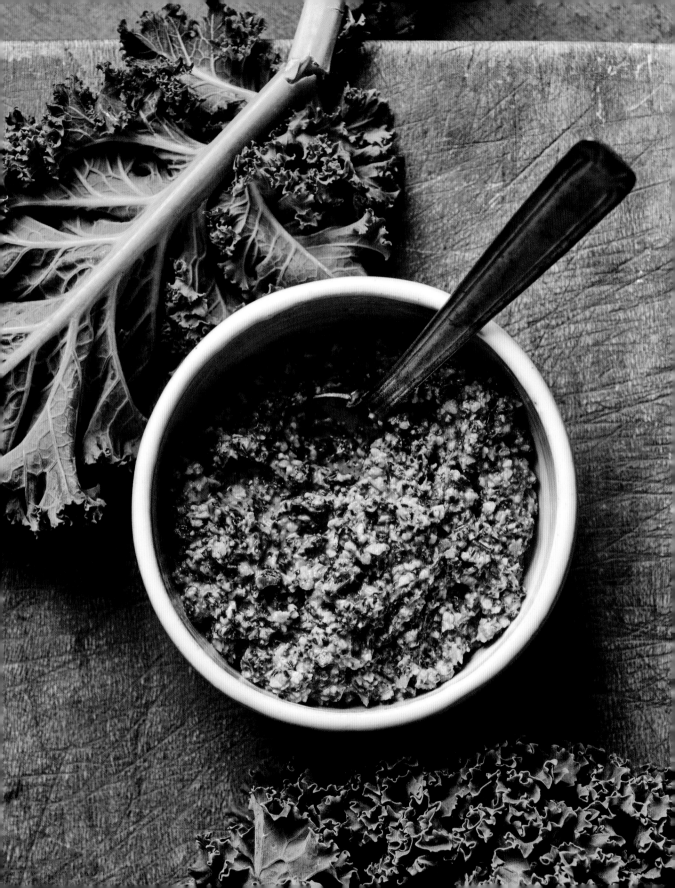

CHAPTER 5

FAKEAWAYS

PINTO BEAN & SWEET POTATO CHILLI

WITH LIME & CORIANDER RICE

This meat-free chilli is inspired by the chilli-chocolate flavours of a Mexican mole. One of my quick Salsas (see pages 162–167) works well with this.

PREP TIME: 7 MINUTES
COOK TIME: 22 MINUTES

spray oil
1 red onion, finely chopped
2 sweet potatoes, peeled and cut
   into small cubes
1 garlic clove, crushed
2 teaspoons balsamic vinegar
300ml (½ pint) hot vegetable stock
300g (10½oz) tomato passata
2 teaspoons honey
2 × 400g (14oz) cans of pinto beans,
   drained and rinsed

FOR THE SPICE MIX
2 teaspoons cocoa powder
1 teaspoon mild chilli powder
½ teaspoon dried oregano
½ teaspoon ground cumin
½ teaspoon ground coriander
¼ teaspoon ground cinnamon
½ teaspoon salt

FOR THE LIME & CORIANDER RICE
300g (10½oz) white basmati rice
finely grated zest and juice of 1 lime
large handful of coriander, finely
   chopped, plus extra to serve

1. Make up the spice mix by mixing all the ingredients in a small bowl.
2. Spray a sauté pan with oil and stir-fry the onion and sweet potatoes for 5 minutes, then stir through the garlic and spice mix and cook for about 30 seconds.
3. Add the balsamic vinegar, give it a stir, then pour in the hot stock and passata.
4. Add the honey and the beans and bring to a simmer, then cook on a medium heat for 15 minutes, stirring occasionally.
5. Meanwhile, cook the rice according to the packet instructions, adding the lime zest to the cooking water.
6. When the rice is cooked and fluffy, drain, then stir in the lime juice and coriander.
7. Serve the rice in warmed bowls, spoon the beans over the top and scatter a little more coriander on top.

NOTE You can mix up the beans in this if you wish: black beans, kidney beans, black-eyed beans, haricot beans, cannellini beans and borlotti beans all work well. The chilli can be frozen, but not the rice.

PER SERVING: Calories 576 | Fat 3.2g | Sat Fat 0.7g | Carbs 111g | Sugars 16g | Fibre 12g | Protein 19g | Salt 1.6g

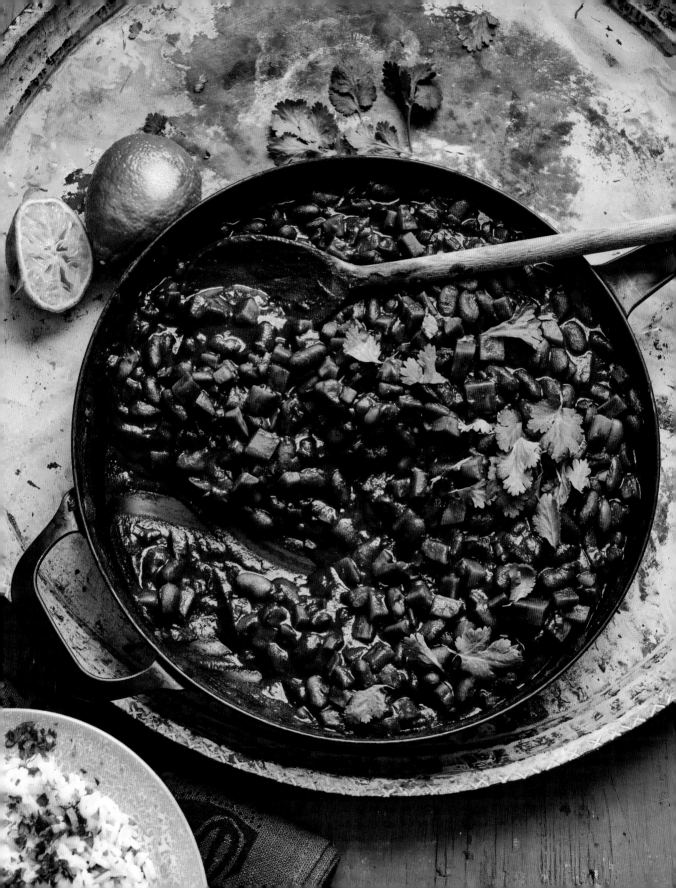

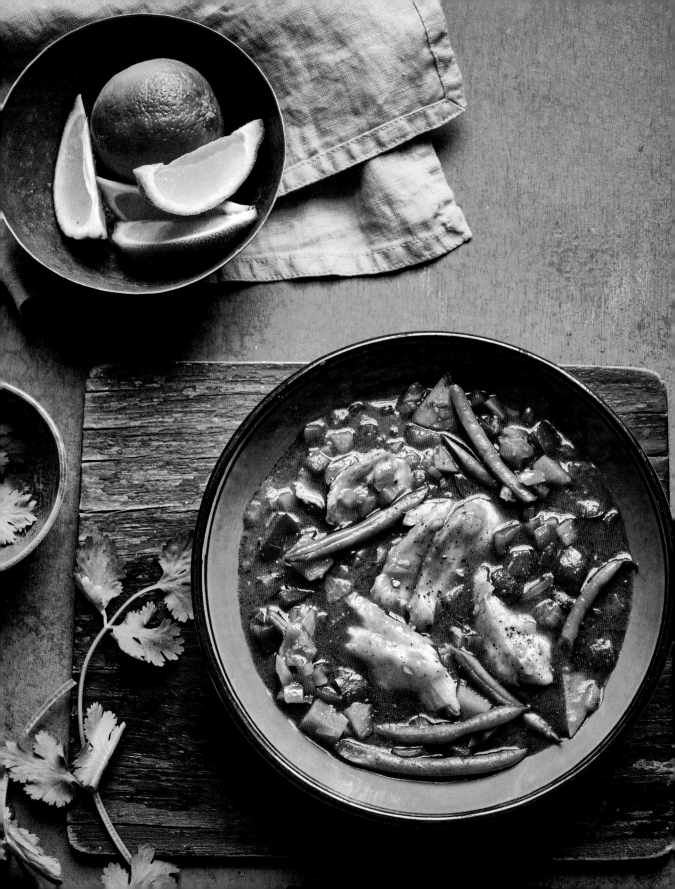

THAI-STYLE RED FISH & SWEET POTATO CURRY

This is one of my favourite quick and easy fakeaways. Simple white fish, steamed on top of the sauce, and tender sweet potato add a different twist. Serve with plain rice, or my Lime & Coriander Rice (see page 136).

PREP TIME: 8 MINUTES

COOK TIME: 20 MINUTES

spray oil

1 onion, finely chopped

1 red pepper, deseeded and finely
   chopped

1 large sweet potato, peeled and
   cut into 1cm (½ inch) cubes

2 tablespoons Thai red curry paste
   (see note)

200ml (7fl oz) chicken stock

400ml (14fl oz) can of light
   coconut milk

250g (9oz) white basmati rice

about 250g (9oz) skinless white
   fish fillet, cut into pieces

100g (3½oz) fine green beans,
   topped, tailed and cut in half

TO SERVE

lime wedges

coriander leaves

1. Spray a sauté pan (for which you have a lid) with oil and fry the onion, red pepper and sweet potato for about 4 minutes, stirring every now and again. Add the red curry paste and stir through for 1 minute.

2. Pour in the stock and coconut milk, stir to combine the sauce, then bring to the boil. Reduce the heat to a simmer and simmer for 10 minutes.

3. Meanwhile, cook the rice according to the packet instructions.

4. When the curry sauce has simmered for 10 minutes, add the fish and green beans, place a lid on the pan and simmer for another 5 minutes or until the fish is cooked. Drain the rice.

5. Try a piece of sweet potato to check that it is cooked through, then serve the curry over the rice with lime wedges and coriander leaves.

NOTE Broccoli, spinach and peas all work well in this dish. Most supermarkets own-brand red curry pastes tend not to be overly spicy. A more authentic brand from an Asian supermarket might have more spice to it, so bear this in mind when adding it – you can always taste the sauce and add more paste. Conversely, if the paste you have is not spicy enough for your taste, you can add extra chilli yourself, either finely chopped fresh chilli or chilli flakes. The curry can be frozen, but not the rice.

PER SERVING: Calories 491 | Fat 8.7g | Sat Fat 6.5g | Carbs 78g | Sugars 12g | Fibre 6.2g | Protein 22g | Salt 1.3g

SPICY TUNA QUESADILLAS

We often turn to quesadillas for a quick lunch or dinner and it only takes a few simple ingredients to make a really satisfying and tasty tuna quesadilla. Serve this with mixed salad or fries.

PREP TIME: 5 MINUTES
COOK TIME: 7 MINUTES

1 roasted red pepper in brine, from a jar, finely sliced
1 spring onion, finely sliced
60g (2¼oz) can of tuna in spring water, drained
4 pickled jalapeño slices, chopped
¼ teaspoon ground cumin
¼ teaspoon chilli flakes
2 large tortillas
60g (2¼oz) red Leicester cheese, grated
salt and pepper, to taste

1. In a bowl, mix together the red pepper, spring onion, tuna, jalapeño, cumin and chilli, then season with salt and pepper.
2. Lay the first tortilla in a cold frying pan, spread the tuna mixture evenly over it and scatter with the cheese. Lay the second tortilla over the top and gently press down to start to stick them together.
3. Put the pan over a high heat for 1 minute, then reduce the heat to medium and cook for 3 minutes.
4. Use a spatula to carefully press down on the top, then flip the quesadilla on to its other side and fry for 3 minutes. Keep an eye on it just to make sure it doesn't start to burn. You want the outside to be golden brown and crispy, and the cheese in the middle to be melted and stick everything together.
5. Remove from the heat and use a sharp knife or pizza cutter to cut it into quarters. Serve with extra spring onion parsley leaves and lime wedges for squeezing over if you like.

NOTE To make a vegetarian version, use a fork to lightly mash a can of black beans or pinto beans and use these to replace the tuna, and make sure your cheese is suitable for vegetarians.

PER SERVING: Calories 384 | Fat 14g | Sat Fat 8.2g | Carbs 41g | Sugars 8.7g | Fibre 4.1g | Protein 21g | Salt 2.4g

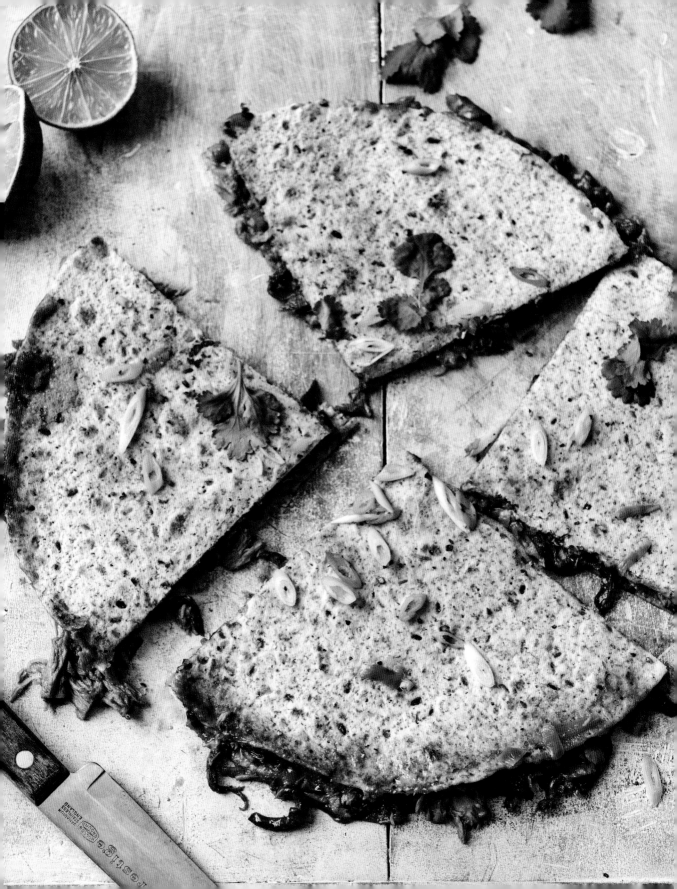

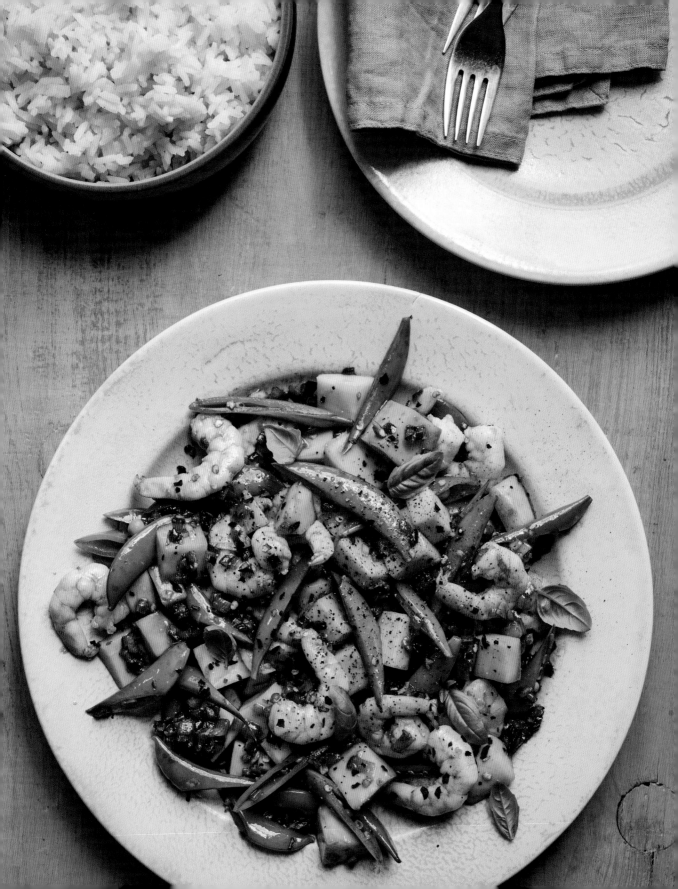

SWEET & SPICY MANGO PRAWNS

A really attractive and delicious dish with tender, sweet mango. I love this simply served with jasmine rice, but it will also work well with noodles.

PREP TIME: 10 MINUTES
COOK TIME: 7 MINUTES

2 garlic cloves, crushed
2 tablespoons light soy sauce
1 tablespoon sweet chilli sauce
juice of 1 lime
spray oil
1 red onion, very finely chopped
165g (5¾oz) raw, peeled king prawns
1 ripe mango, chopped into 2cm (¾ inch) cubes (see note for how to prepare a mango)
100g (3½oz) sugarsnap peas, topped and tailed

TO SERVE
basil leaves, torn
freshly ground black pepper

1. In a small bowl, mix together the garlic, soy sauce, sweet chilli sauce and lime juice.
2. Spray a frying pan or sauté pan with oil and sauté the onion for 3 minutes, then stir in the sauce from the bowl.
3. Add the king prawns and stir-fry until pink (about 2 minutes), then add the mango and sugarsnap peas and stir-fry over a high heat for 2 more minutes.
4. Serve, tearing basil leaves over the top and with a few grinds of black pepper.

> **HOW TO PREPARE A MANGO**
> Stand the mango on a chopping board with the stem end facing upwards and the 'cheeks' (the fatter fleshy parts) to either side. Using a sharp knife, slice down about 1cm (½ inch) away from the stem all the way to the bottom; if you hit the stone in the middle, just gently guide the knife around it and keep cutting downwards until you have removed the first cheek. Repeat on the other side. You can use the knife to score a cross-hatch pattern through the flesh but not piercing the skin. You should then be able to turn the skin inside out. Use a sharp-edged spoon, or small paring knife, to remove the chunks of mango from the skin. For the flesh around the stone, you can either use a knife to shave away any flesh, or the easier option is just to pick it up and eat what's left around the stone.

PER SERVING: Calories 226 | Fat 1.4g | Sat Fat 0.4g | Carbs 32g | Sugars 30g | Fibre 1.4g | Protein 18.6g | Salt 2.8g

SPICY PRAWN FISHCAKES
WITH A SWEET CHILLI & LIME DIP

These little fishcakes are incredibly simple to make, but packed with amazing Thai-inspired flavours. This is a recipe where you do need to use sesame oil for frying: it contributes to the flavour and allows the fishcakes to hold together, as well as to not stick to the pan. These go really well with crisp vegetable sides, such as shredded cabbage and carrot, crunchy salads or stir-fried vegetables, but also noodles or rice.

PREP TIME: 10 MINUTES
COOK TIME: 9–18 MINUTES

150g (5½oz) cooked, peeled
   cold-water prawns
280g (10oz) skinless white
   fish fillets
2 tablespoons Thai red curry paste
   (see page 139)
4 spring onions, trimmed
large handful of coriander
1 red chilli, deseeded and roughly
   chopped
finely grated zest of 1 lime
1 tablespoon fish sauce
1 egg yolk (see page 221 for how to
   separate eggs)
½ teaspoon salt
70g (2½oz) fine green beans,
   topped and tailed, and roughly
   chopped
1 tablespoon toasted sesame oil

FOR THE DIPPING SAUCE
4 tablespoons sweet chilli sauce
juice of 1 lime

1. Put everything except the green beans, sesame oil and dipping sauce ingredients in a food processor and blend until finely chopped.

2. Add the green beans, then blend again until the mixture is very finely blended and the green beans are well chopped.

3. Put the sesame oil into a large, cold frying pan and spread it around to cover the bottom. I make the fishcakes and put them directly into the pan, as they are a fairly wet mixture and this method saves having to handle them too much. (You may need to cook them in 2 batches, depending on the size of your pan.)

4. To make the fishcakes, wet your hands, then use your palms to form 12 patties, each about 4cm (1½ inches) in diameter, then place in the oiled pan.

5. Once you have all the fishcakes (or half the batch) in the pan, put it over a high heat and fry for 5 minutes. Flip the fishcakes over and fry on the other side for 4 minutes. Remove from the pan and repeat the process if you have more to cook (there should be enough residual oil in the pan for this).

6. In a small bowl, mix the sweet chilli sauce with the lime juice until combined, then serve with the fishcakes.

NOTE Use any the leftover egg white to make my Oat, Chickpea & Herb Crackers (see page 196).

PER SERVING: Calories 174 | Fat 2.7g | Sat Fat 0.6g | Carbs 14g | Sugars 12g | Fibre 1.8g | Protein 22g | Salt 2.3g

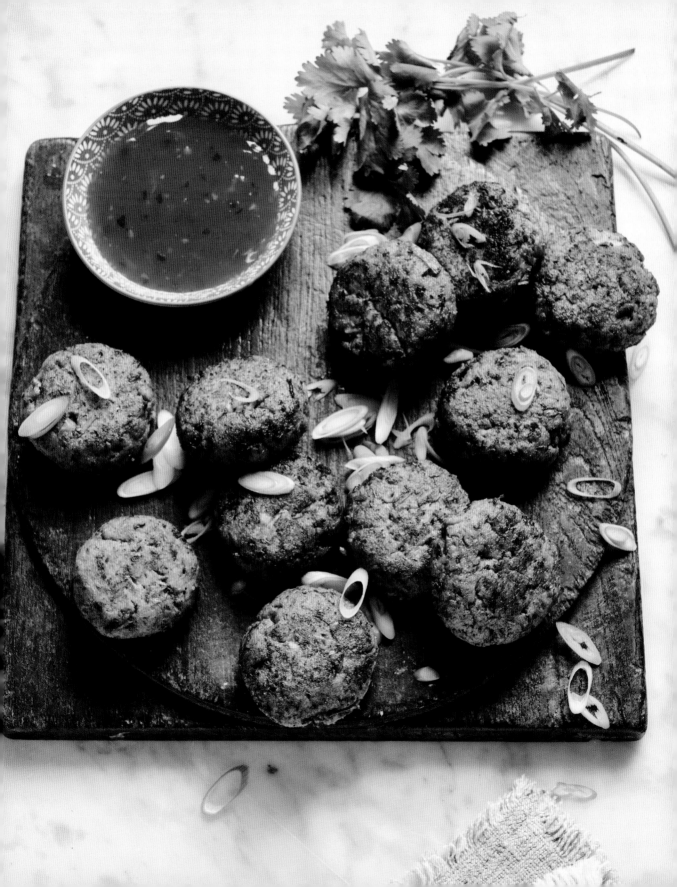

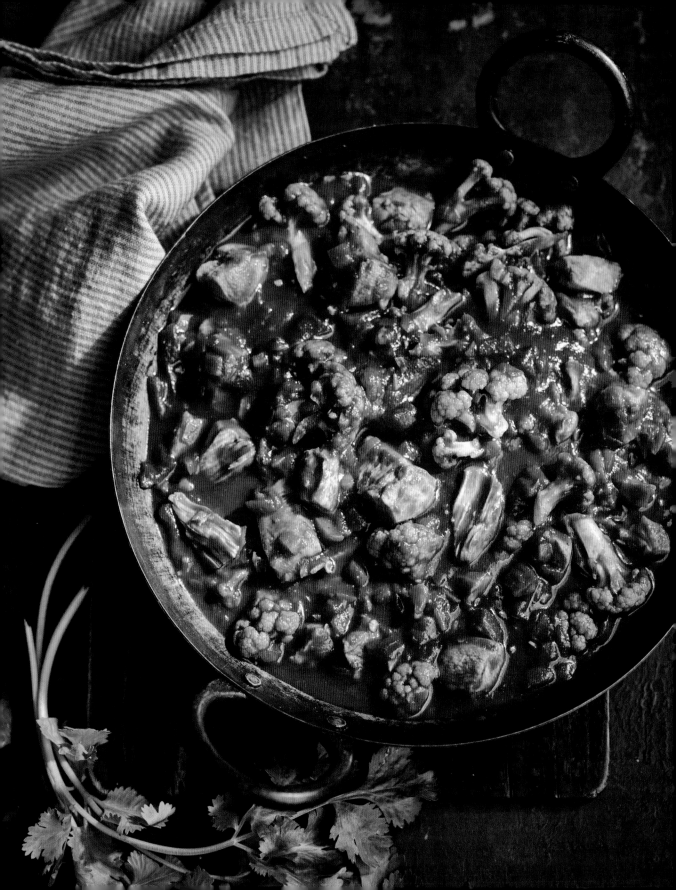

WARMING CHICKEN & CAULIFLOWER CURRY

A satisfyingly saucy curry that only uses really simple ingredients, as well as curry powder instead of multiple spices. This is a perfect curry-in-a-hurry, which you can either serve alongside rice, or with simple steamed green vegetables such as Tenderstem broccoli or green beans.

PREP TIME: 8 MINUTES
COOK TIME: 20 MINUTES

spray oil
1 onion, finely chopped
3 garlic cloves, crushed
1 chilli (green or red), deseeded and
    finely chopped
3 skinless chicken breasts,
    chopped into bite-sized pieces
2 tablespoons mild curry powder
500g (1lb 2oz) tomato passata
200ml (7fl oz) chicken stock
2 roasted red peppers in brine,
    from a jar (about 160g / 5¾oz)
    drained and chopped
½ cauliflower, chopped into bite-
    sized florets
1 teaspoon salt
½ teaspoon pepper
coriander leaves, to serve (optional)

1. Spray a sauté pan or deep frying pan (for which you have a lid) with oil and stir-fry the onion, garlic, green chilli and chicken over a high heat for 5 minutes.

2. Stir the curry powder through for 30 seconds, then add the passata, stock and red peppers. Reduce the heat to medium and simmer for 5 minutes.

3. Add the cauliflower, salt and pepper, stir them into the sauce, pop a lid on the pan and simmer gently for 5 minutes.

4. Remove the lid from the pan and simmer for a further 5 minutes, then check the chicken is cooked through (see page 109).

5. Serve with some coriander scattered on top, if you like.

NOTE You can add extras to the sauce if you want to bulk this up or increase the amount of vegetables: try frozen peas, chopped courgette, green beans or chickpeas added at the same time as the cauliflower. If you wish to change the protein in the curry, you could switch the chicken for prawns or white fish (rather than frying with the onion, add these at the same time as the passata). To make this vegetarian, substitute the chicken for chickpeas and canned lentils (add these with the passata) and switch the chicken stock for vegetable stock.

PER SERVING: Calories 202 | Fat 2.7g | Sat Fat 0.6g | Carbs 18g | Sugars 13g | Fibre 5.9g | Protein 24g | Salt 2.4g

147 | FAKEAWAYS

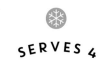

SPICY BASIL CHICKEN

One of my favourite ways to use minced chicken... This dish is spicy, aromatic and savoury with just a touch of sweetness. Thai basil isn't always easy to get hold of in the UK, but this still tastes great using regular basil. We serve it in lettuce wraps or pitta bread, sometimes a Thai-style coleslaw, but it also goes really well with rice or noodles, and is great topped off with a fried egg.

PREP TIME: 10 MINUTES
COOK TIME: 10 MINUTES

spray oil
4 shallots, finely chopped
4 garlic cloves, crushed
1 bird's eye chilli, deseeded and
   finely chopped (see note)
500g (1lb 2oz) lean minced chicken
2 tablespoons dark soy sauce
1 tablespoon fish sauce
1 teaspoon honey
large handful of basil leaves,
   roughly shredded
lime wedges, to serve

1. Spray a sauté pan with oil and sauté the shallots, garlic and chilli over a medium heat for 1 minute. Add the minced chicken, increase the heat to high and stir-fry for 4 minutes, using a wooden spoon to break down any clumps as you cook.

2. Add the soy sauce, fish sauce and honey, reduce the heat to medium once more and continue to stir-fry for another 5 minutes.

3. Remove from the heat and stir the shredded basil through the chicken. Serve with lime wedges if you like.

NOTE Bird's eye chillies are available in most supermarkets. They are small, thin and pointy and usually come in a mix of green and red. They pack a great intense heat and have a fruity flavour. You can eat them with or without the seeds (which are extra-spicy). I have suggested 1 chilli in this recipe, but if you love a real spicy kick then you can use more. Equally, if you are cautious around spicy food, you can always just add half to start with and stir in more at the end if you want a bit more heat.

PER SERVING: Calories 176 | Fat 2.6g | Sat Fat 0.8g | Carbs 6.1g | Sugars 5.1g | Fibre 1.3g | Protein 31g | Salt 2.5g

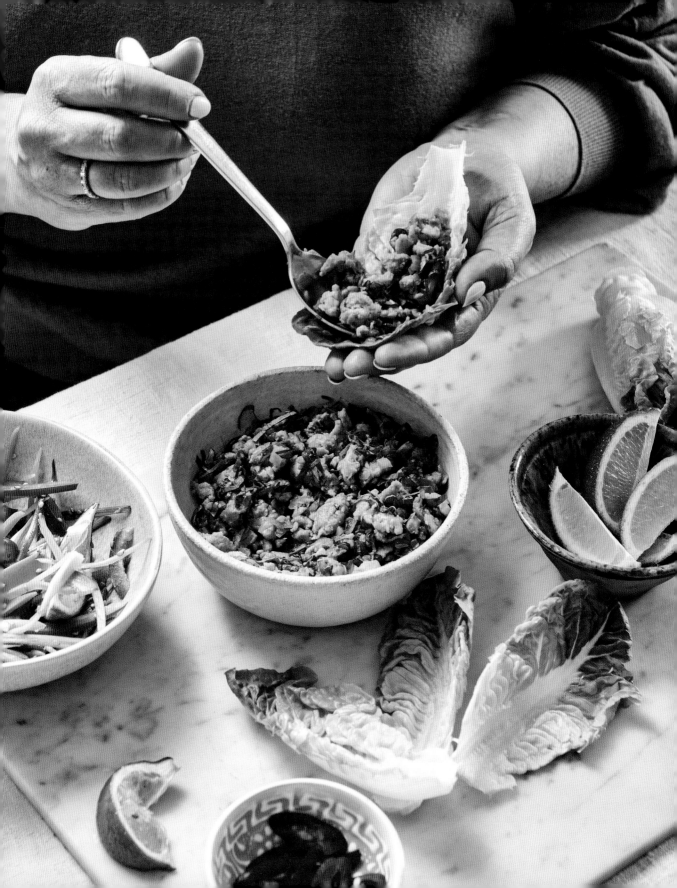

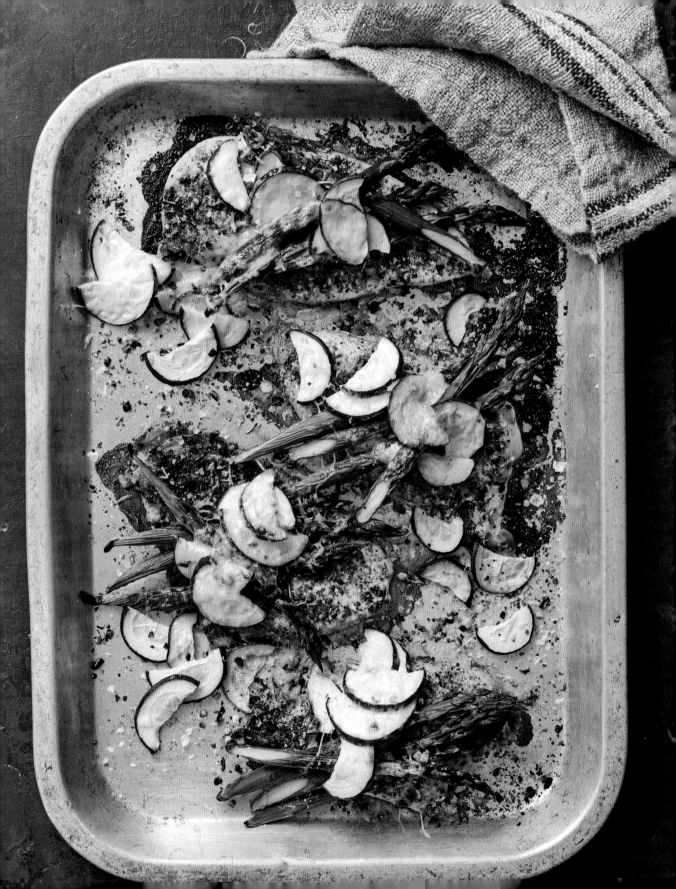

PERI-PERI CHICKEN CHEDDAR BAKE

So simple to make, but so satisfying to eat. I make up peri-peri spice mix in batches so that I have it ready for quick meals (see note, below), but most supermarkets now sell their own version of peri-peri seasoning if you haven't had a chance to make your own. I usually serve this with a mixed salad, but you could also serve it with fries or potato wedges.

PREP TIME: 5 MINUTES

COOK TIME: 25 MINUTES

2 chicken breasts, sliced in half horizontally
1 tablespoon peri-peri spice mix (see note)
16 asparagus spears, woody ends trimmed away
1 courgette, sliced
finely grated zest and juice of 1 lemon
60g (2¼oz) Cheddar cheese, grated

1. Preheat the oven to 220°C/200°C fan (425°F), Gas Mark 7.
2. Spread the chicken breast halves out flat in a small casserole dish or flameproof oven dish.
3. Sprinkle over the peri-peri seasoning, then arrange the vegetables on top of the breasts.
4. Pour over the lemon juice, sprinkle over the zest, then scatter the cheese over the vegetables.
5. Bake for 20 minutes or until the chicken is cooked through (see page 109), making sure you preheat the grill for the last 5 minutes. Move the dish to under the grill and grill the top for 5 minutes to ensure the cheese is golden-brown and bubbling.

> **TO MAKE YOUR OWN PERI-PERI SPICE MIX**
> Simply combine all the following ingredients in a jam jar or other airtight container. It will keep for up to 6 months.
> **1 tablespoon each of** sweet paprika; onion granules; garlic granules; sugar or granulated sweetener; ground coriander; chilli flakes, **plus 1½ teaspoons each of** salt; pepper; dried parsley; dried oregano; cayenne pepper and ground cumin.

PER SERVING: Calories 343 | Fat 14g | Sat Fat 7.3g | Carbs 5.4g | Sugars 5.2g | Fibre 3.4g | Protein 45g | Salt 1.1g

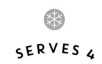

BRISK BUTTER CHICKEN

This is not an authentic butter chicken, but rather my interpretation of it, using my favourite key flavours as a quick solution to making a creamy, satisfying and slightly indulgent curry. I love to have lots of sauce, so this recipe does, and I also really think you need butter and cream to truly make it special. Just using the small amounts in this recipe gives beautiful flavour and creaminess. I serve this simply with white basmati rice scattered with coriander, or Turmeric Rice (see page 208).

PREP TIME: 5 MINUTES

COOK TIME: 22 MINUTES

4 skinless chicken breasts (total weight about 800g / 1lb 12oz), cut into chunks

1 teaspoon ground cinnamon

1 teaspoon sweet paprika

1 tablespoon melted unsalted butter

spray oil

1 onion, finely chopped

1 teaspoon garlic paste

1 teaspoon ginger paste

1 teaspoon garam masala

1 teaspoon ground fenugreek seeds

1 teaspoon ground turmeric

1 teaspoon chilli powder

500g (1lb 2oz) tomato passata

200ml (7fl oz) hot chicken stock

1 teaspoon sugar

1 teaspoon salt

100ml (3½fl oz) single cream

2 teaspoons cornflour

coriander leaves, to serve

1. Preheat the oven to 240°C/220°C fan (475°F), Gas Mark 9.
2. In a deep baking tray, mix the chicken breast chunks with the cinnamon, paprika and melted butter and place into the oven for 20 minutes.
3. Meanwhile, spray a sauté pan with oil and gently fry the onion for 5 minutes to soften it, then stir through the garlic and ginger pastes, then the garam masala, fenugreek, turmeric and chilli powder. Stir-fry for 30 seconds. Add the passata, hot stock, sugar and salt and leave to simmer for 15 minutes.
4. Remove the chicken from the oven and stir it through the sauce. Pour in the cream, then separately mix the cornflour in a small bowl with a little bit of cold water until it is a smooth liquid. Stir this into the sauce.
5. Simmer the sauce for another 2 minutes, stirring it constantly until it has thickened before serving with coriander leaves scattered on top.

NOTE Sometimes I like to bulk out my butter chicken with some extra vegetables and I often use butternut squash. You could roast this in the oven at the same time as the chicken, using frozen butternut squash cubes for ease: simply spray them with oil and roast for about 20 minutes alongside the chicken, before mixing both into the sauce.

PER SERVING: Calories 320 | Fat 11g | Sat Fat 5.8g | Carbs 15g | Sugars 9.6g | Fibre 3.8g | Protein 38g | Salt 2.6g

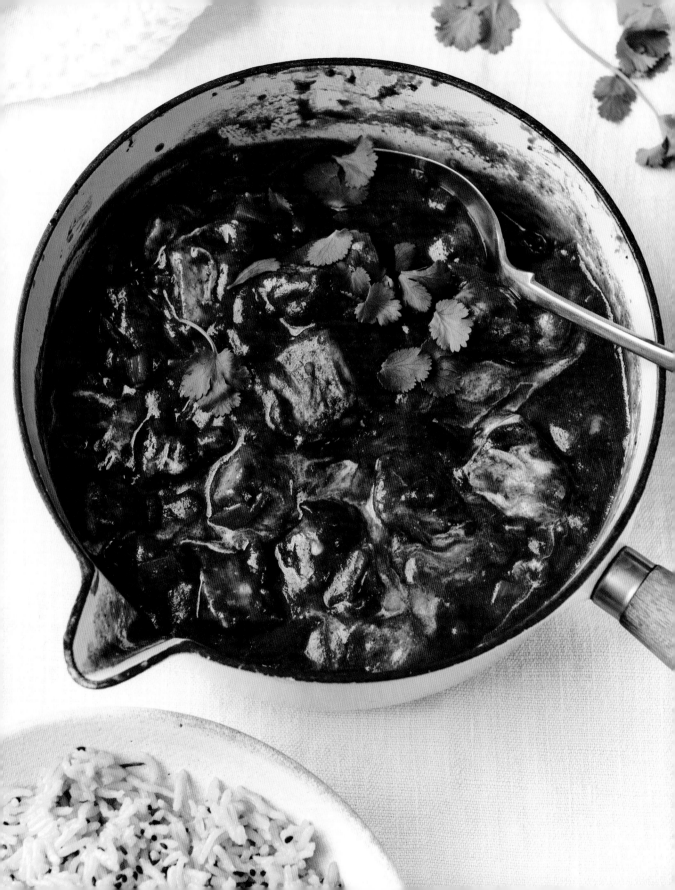

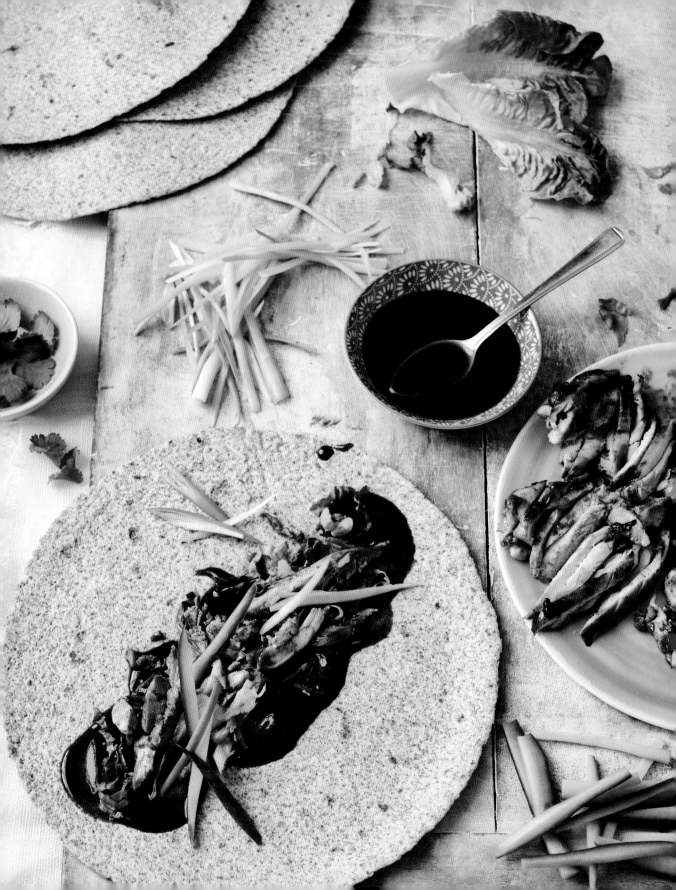

HOISIN CHICKEN WRAPS

I've always loved crispy duck pancakes and this is a cheat's version
that is cheaper, quicker and leaner: you still get some of the great
key flavours, but without much hard work. It's up to you whether you
want to make your own hoisin sauce (see page 61), as hoisin is readily
available to buy and the wraps will still taste great.

PREP TIME: 5 MINUTES
COOK TIME: 20 MINUTES

8 skinless chicken thigh fillets,
   excess fat trimmed away
2 tablespoons hoisin sauce, plus
   extra for the wraps
spray oil
4 tortilla wraps
1 Little Gem lettuce, shredded
½ cucumber, cut into matchsticks
6 spring onions, finely sliced
   lengthways

1. Preheat the oven to 240°C/220°C fan (475°F), Gas Mark 9.
2. Splay the chicken thigh fillets open and place them on a
   baking tray, then spread the 2 tablespoons hoisin sauce
   over to cover and spray lightly with oil.
3. Bake for 20 minutes, turning them over halfway through.
4. Check the chicken is cooked through (see page 109).
   Allow to rest for 5 minutes, then finely slice the thighs
   with a sharp knife.
5. Spread a little hoisin sauce on the inside of each wrap,
   then add shredded lettuce, cooked chicken, cucumber
   and spring onions before wrapping. Or just put all the
   elements on the table and let everyone do their own.

NOTE This is a light meal on its own and you may wish to
add extra sides. I use tortillas as it can be hard to get hold of
Chinese pancakes, but if you can find those then use them
instead. You can also use mini tortillas for young children.

PER SERVING: Calories 441 | Fat 16g | Sat Fat 4.9g | Carbs 38g | Sugars 5.5g | Fibre 3.9g | Protein 35g | Salt 1.3g

KOREAN-STYLE STICKY CHILLI CHICKEN

After having a version of this from a takeaway, my husband and I were addicted. My husband usually makes it by deep-frying the chicken to get it crispy, but my baked version is just as satisfying. By crisping the chicken up with a little cornflour in the oven, and using Korean-style flavours in the sticky sauce, this hits the spot at a fraction of the calories. Serve with jasmine rice.

PREP TIME: 5 MINUTES
COOK TIME: 25 MINUTES

6 skinless chicken thigh fillets, excess fat trimmed away, each cut into 6
3 tablespoons cornflour
low-calorie cooking spray
2 spring onions, sliced, to serve

FOR THE STICKY SAUCE
2 garlic cloves, crushed
2cm (¾ inch) piece of fresh root ginger, peeled and finely grated
2 tablespoons dark soy sauce
2 tablespoons honey
1 tablespoon rice wine
1 tablespoon gochujang paste (see note)
1 tablespoon apple cider vinegar
1 tablespoon soft dark brown sugar
1 teaspoon toasted sesame oil

1. Preheat the oven to 220°C/200°C fan (425°F), Gas Mark 7.
2. Place the chicken pieces in a bowl and sprinkle over the cornflour, then mix until it is fairly evenly coated.
3. Line a large baking tray with nonstick baking paper, spray it with low-calorie cooking spray, then lay the chicken pieces on the paper, leaving a gap between each one. Spray the chicken generously with cooking spray, then place in the oven for 25 minutes or until cooked through.
4. Meanwhile, make the sticky sauce. Put all the ingredients in a small pan and stir them together. Place over a low heat and cook gently, stirring occasionally, until you have a smooth, thick sauce. Allow to simmer for 10 minutes and then set aside until the chicken is ready.
5. When the chicken comes out of the oven it should be tender in the middle and a little crispy on the outside, with some extra-crispy edges. Pop the sauce back over the heat to reheat, then move the chicken from the baking tray into a bowl and pour over the hot, sticky sauce. Mix it thoroughly and serve with sliced spring onions scattered on top.

NOTE Gochujang is a Korean fermented spicy red chilli paste, with an intense sweet-hot-salty flavour, and is now available in most supermarkets. If you buy some it won't go to waste – try it in the recipes on pages 182 and 198.

PER SERVING: Calories 316 | Fat 13g | Sat Fat 3.2g | Carbs 29g | Sugars 14g | Fibre 0.5g | Protein 21g | Salt 2g

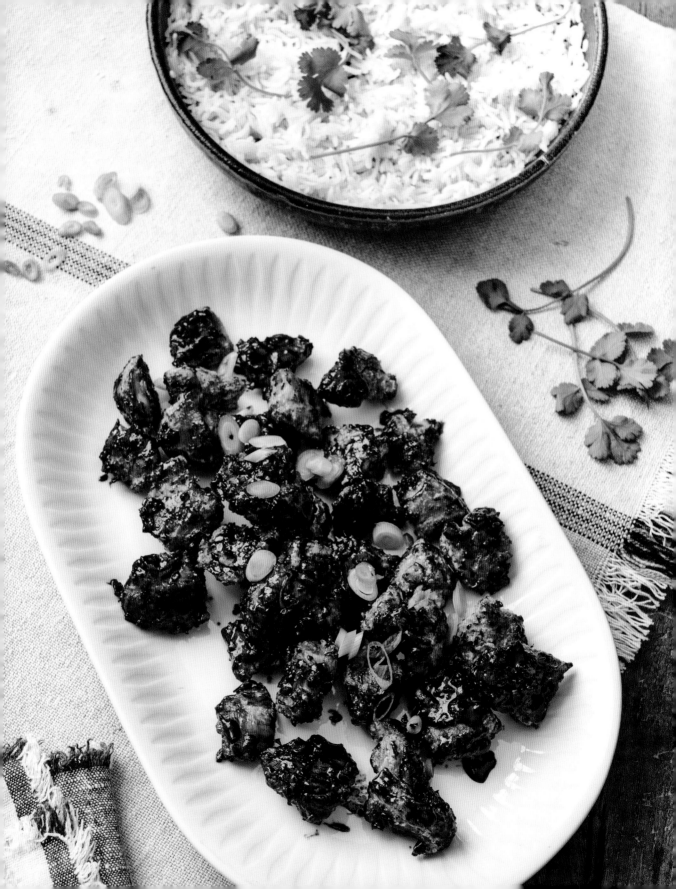

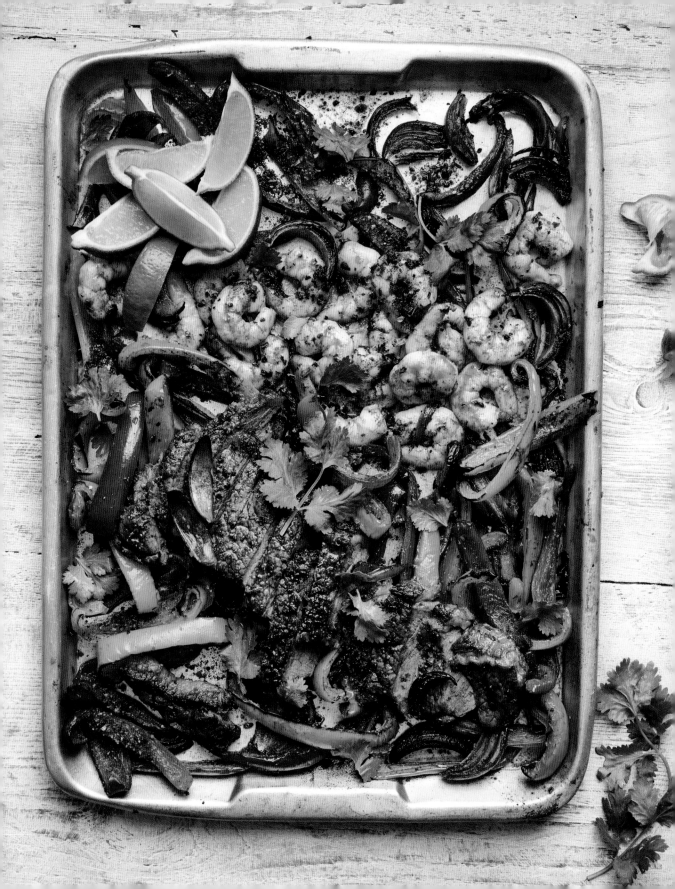

SURF 'N' TURF FAJITA TRAYBAKE

This combination of steak and prawns in fajitas is an indulgent but delicious mix, perfect for a treat. I prefer to buy a good cut of steak to avoid unpleasantly chewy meat. By cooking the steak whole, then allowing it time to rest, you should achieve melt-in-the-mouth meat. Serve this mix in wraps (with lettuce, refried beans, salsa and grated cheese), or simply serve it with rice (try my Lime & Coriander Rice, see page 136).

PREP TIME: 10 MINUTES

COOK TIME: 20 MINUTES

spray oil

2 sirloin or ribeye steaks (total weight 400–500g / 14oz–1lb 2oz)

2 red onions, halved, then finely sliced

4 peppers (a mix of orange, red and yellow), deseeded and cut into strips

150g (5½oz) cooked, peeled king prawns

FOR THE SPICE MIX

½ teaspoon chilli flakes

1 teaspoon smoked paprika

½ teaspoon garlic granules

½ teaspoon onion granules

1 teaspoon dried oregano

1 teaspoon salt

TO SERVE

handful of coriander leaves

lime wedges

1. Preheat the oven to 200°C/180°C fan (400°F), Gas Mark 6.
2. Spray a large baking tray with a little oil and lay the steaks in the centre.
3. For the spice mix, simply mix all the ingredients together in a large bowl.
4. Arrange the onions and peppers around the steaks, then sprinkle the spice mix over everything. Spray the top lightly with oil, then place in the oven and cook for 15 minutes.
5. Remove the tray from the oven and lift the steaks on to a plate to rest. Add the prawns to the baking tray, give everything a stir, then pop the tray back into the oven for 5 minutes.
6. Use a sharp knife to finely slice the steaks. Remove the tray from the oven, then mix the sliced steak back into the fajita mix.
7. Serve scattered with coriander leaves and with lime wedges on the side.

NOTE These cooking times should produce a medium-rare steak, though the size and thickness of the steak will affect this. If you want to bulk this meal out, add some drained canned beans, such as black beans or pinto beans, at the same time as the prawns.

PER SERVING: Calories 350 | Fat 14g | Sat Fat 5.7g | Carbs 14g | Sugars 11g | Fibre 4.9g | Protein 39g | Salt 1.9g

STEAK WITH RED WINE & MUSHROOM SAUCE

Red wine sauce has always been my favourite steak accompaniment. This version is thick and rich, with tasty little button mushrooms adding a little side of veg. My favourite side dishes for this are baby potatoes and asparagus, or homemade fries or sweet potato wedges and peas.

PREP TIME: 5 MINUTES
COOK TIME: 10 MINUTES

1 tablespoon unsalted butter
2 good-quality ribeye or sirloin
   steaks, each 200–250g (7–9oz)
2 shallots, finely chopped
2 garlic cloves, crushed
100ml (3½fl oz) red wine
200g (7oz) baby button
   mushrooms
100ml (3½fl oz) beef stock
½ teaspoon Dijon mustard
1 teaspoon cornflour
1 tablespoon cold water
salt and pepper, to taste

1. Put the butter in a frying pan over a high heat and swirl it around to cover the bottom of the pan as it melts (or use a silicone pastry brush to distribute it).
2. Lay both the steaks in the pan. Keep the heat high and fry for 2 minutes on each side for medium-rare (or longer if you like it more well done).
3. Remove the steaks to a plate, season them with salt and pepper and leave to rest while you make the sauce. (If you want to warm the plate first, then you can do so under the grill or in the oven.)
4. Place the steak pan back over a medium heat and add the shallots and garlic. Stir these for 20–30 seconds until you can just smell the garlic (you want to ensure that the garlic does not burn, so have the wine ready), then pour in the red wine and quickly stir it through, allowing it to bubble vigorously for 1 minute.
5. Add the mushrooms to the pan, then the stock and mustard. Stir to combine, then simmer for 2 minutes.
6. Prepare the cornflour by dissolving it in the cold water until you have a smooth liquid, then add it to the sauce. Allow the sauce to simmer for another 3 minutes, stirring occasionally while it thickens.
7. Slice the steaks and arrange them on warmed plates. Spoon over the sauce and serve with side dishes of your choice.

PER SERVING: Calories 509 | Fat 25g | Sat Fat 12g | Carbs 9.2g | Sugars 3.1g | Fibre 3.3g | Protein 52g | Salt 1g

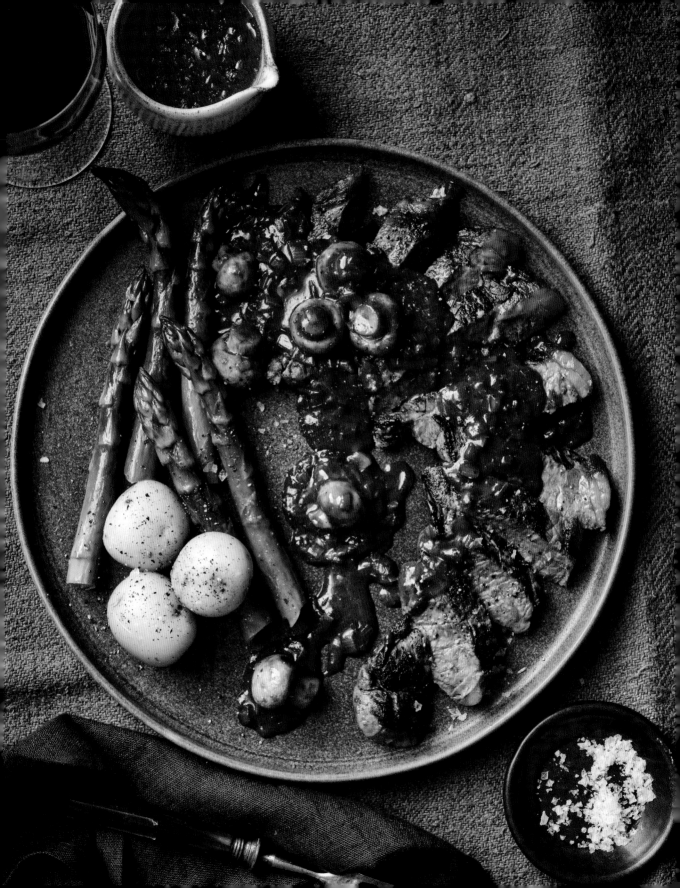

3 WAYS WITH SALSA

Salsas are handy condiments that can really liven up a meal. They make a great fancy touch at barbecues and other get-togethers, while also adding extra veg.

SERVES 4

DARK & SMOKY CHIPOTLE SALSA

This salsa is saucy, similar to the jars of salsa you can buy, with rich, smoky flavour. Perfect as a dip, as a side, in burrito bowls, with tacos, fajitas or nachos.

PREP TIME: 5 MINUTES
COOK TIME: 25 MINUTES

2 onions, finely chopped
spray oil
3 garlic cloves, crushed
1 tablespoon balsamic vinegar
400g (14oz) can of chopped
    tomatoes
1 teaspoon chipotle chilli flakes
1 teaspoon smoked paprika
½ teaspoon salt
1 teaspoon honey
small handful of coriander
    leaves and stalks, finely
    chopped, plus extra to serve

1. Fry the onions in spray oil for 5 minutes, then stir through the garlic.
2. Add the balsamic vinegar, stir it through the onions, then add the chopped tomatoes, chilli flakes, smoked paprika, salt and honey.
3. Simmer for 20 minutes, stirring occasionally, then stir in the coriander. Serve hot or cold scattered with extra chopped coriander. If you are setting this aside to serve it cold, just give it a stir before serving.

PER SERVING: Calories 83 | Fat 0.7g | Sat Fat 0g | Carbs 13g | Sugars 11g | Fibre 3.4g | Protein 3g | Salt 0.86g

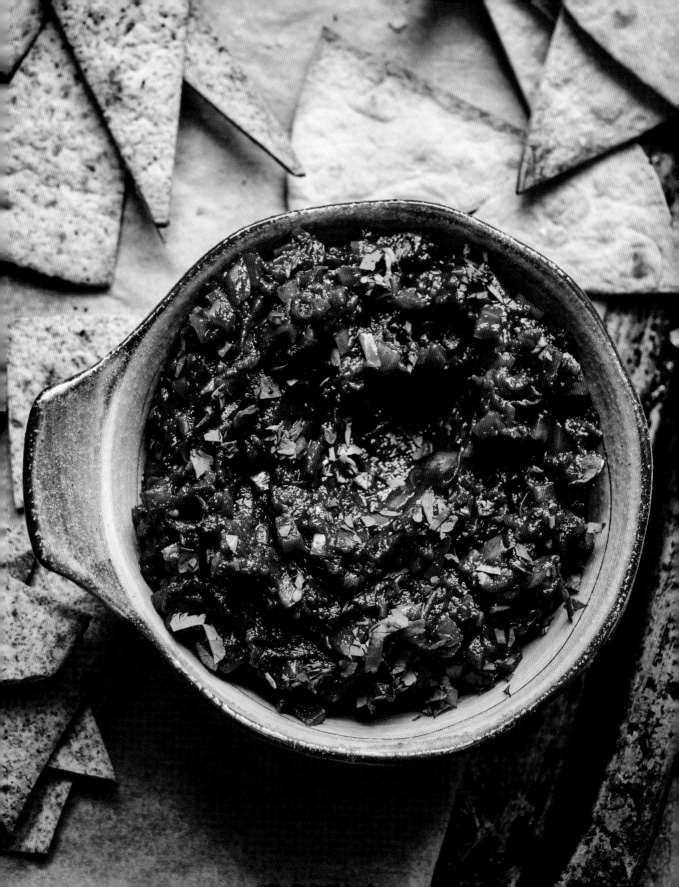

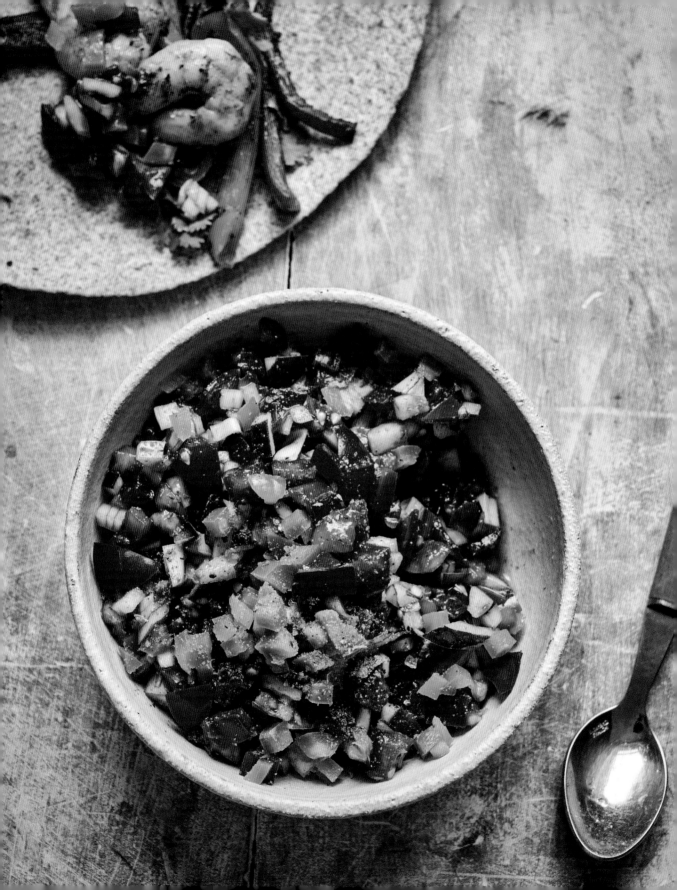

SALSA FRESCA

This is the type of salsa that I ate most frequently when I was in Mexico: a quick combination of finely chopped onion, tomatoes, chillies, coriander and lime. Because our supermarket tomatoes in the UK can be a little insipid, I add some extra flavours to my version, but this is still super-quick to make and a versatile side dish. It's worth spending a little bit of time to chop the ingredients nice and small. You can use a mini chopper, but it will be more liquid and messier this way, as it pulls out a lot of the juice from the tomatoes.

PREP TIME: 12 MINUTES

COOK TIME: NONE

1 red onion, finely chopped
6 salad tomatoes, finely chopped
small handful (about 40g /
    1½oz) pickled jalapeños,
    finely chopped
30g (1oz) coriander, finely
    chopped
¾ teaspoon coarse salt
¼ teaspoon coarsely ground
    black pepper
¼ teaspoon dried oregano
¼ teaspoon ground cumin
juice of 1 lime

1. Once all the ingredients are prepared, simply stir them all together and serve.

PER SERVING: Calories 31 | Fat 0g | Sat Fat 0g | Carbs 5.2g | Sugars 3.3g | Fibre 1.2g | Protein 0.8g | Salt 1.1g

COOLING GREEN APPLE & CUCUMBER SALSA

This is a refreshing salsa that is great for offsetting the spice of another dish and works really well for summer barbecues, or served with simply cooked fish.

PREP TIME: 12 MINUTES
COOK TIME: NONE

2 green apples, such as Granny
    Smith, peeled, cored and
    finely chopped
¼ cucumber, finely chopped
3 spring onions, finely sliced
1 green chilli, deseeded and
    finely chopped
small handful of mint leaves,
    finely chopped
juice of 1 lime
½ teaspoon salt

1. Once all the ingredients are prepared, simply stir them all together and serve.

PER SERVING: Calories 57 | Fat 0.7g | Sat Fat 0g | Carbs 10g | Sugars 9.2g | Fibre 1.5g | Protein 1.3g | Salt 0.62g

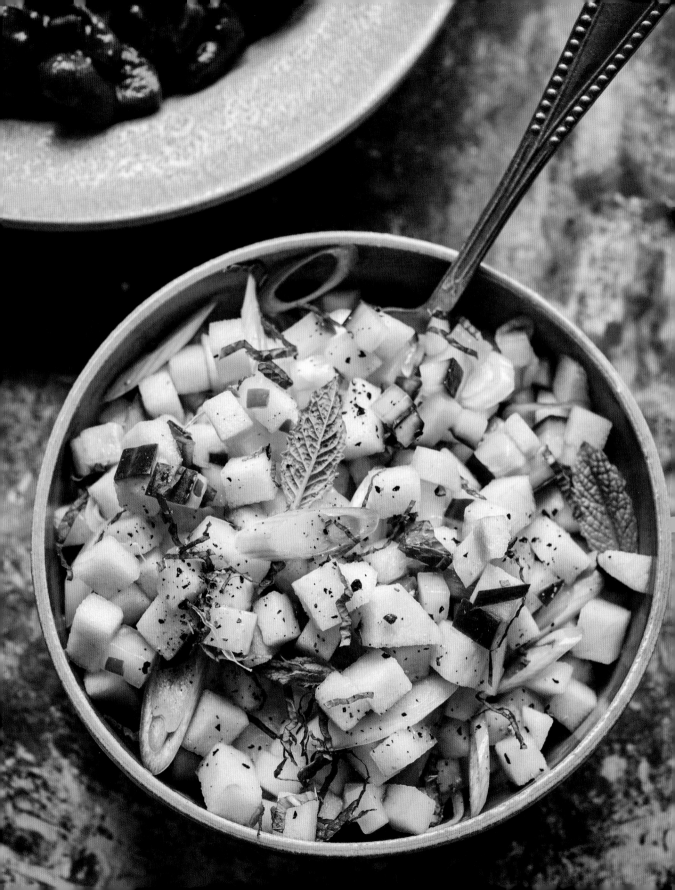

CHAPTER 6

SLAM-DUNK DINNERS

SWEET POTATO, BROCCOLI, COCONUT & QUINOA CURRY

This is a hearty curry with the added filling power of quinoa. Perfect bowl food with no need to cook additional sides unless you want to! I like to serve this with some naan and mango chutney or aubergine pickle on the side.

PREP TIME: 5 MINUTES

COOK TIME: 4–5 HOURS (HIGH) OR 6–8 HOURS (LOW)

1 onion, finely chopped

2 garlic cloves, crushed

5cm (2 inch) piece of fresh root ginger, peeled and finely grated

1 sweet potato (about 250g / 9oz), peeled and chopped into about 1.5cm/½ inch sized cubes

1 head of broccoli, cut into florets

400g (14oz) can of chopped tomatoes

400ml (14fl oz) can of light coconut milk

250ml (9fl oz) vegetable stock

1 tablespoon light soy sauce

40g (1½oz) quinoa (I use mixed colour, but any type is fine)

2 teaspoons ground turmeric

2 teaspoons mustard seeds

1 teaspoon chilli flakes

1 teaspoon salt

1. Put all the ingredients in the slow-cooker pot and give everything a stir.
2. Cook on high for 4–5 hours, or on low for 6–8 hours before serving.

NOTE To cook this in a regular oven, preheat the oven to 200°C/180°C fan (400°F), Gas Mark 6. Put all the ingredients in a casserole dish, place the lid on and cook for 1 hour.

PER SERVING: Calories 191 | Fat 6.6g | Sat Fat 4.4g | Carbs 22g | Sugars 10g | Fibre 6.2g | Protein 7.2g | Salt 1.7g

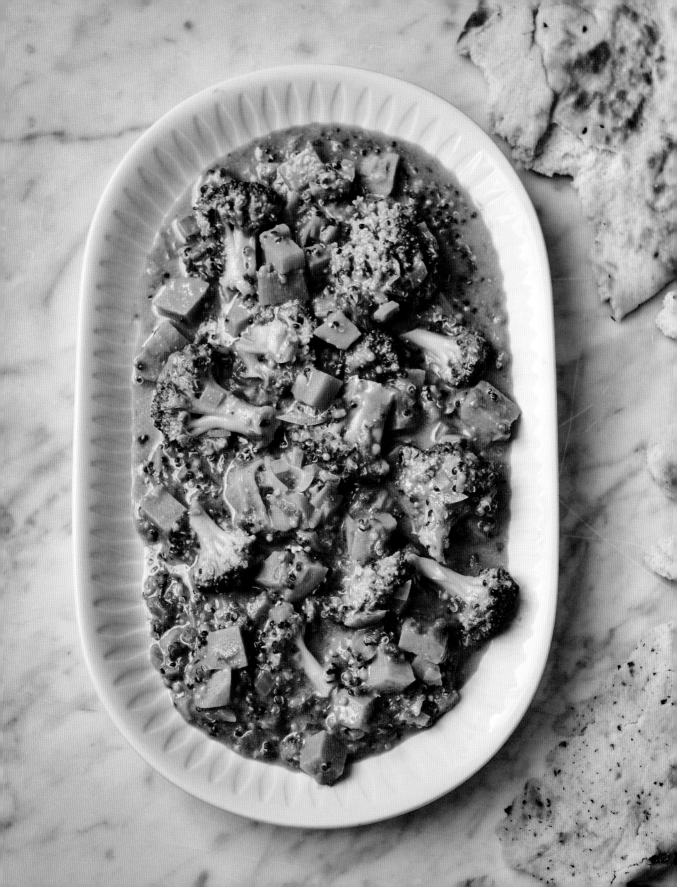

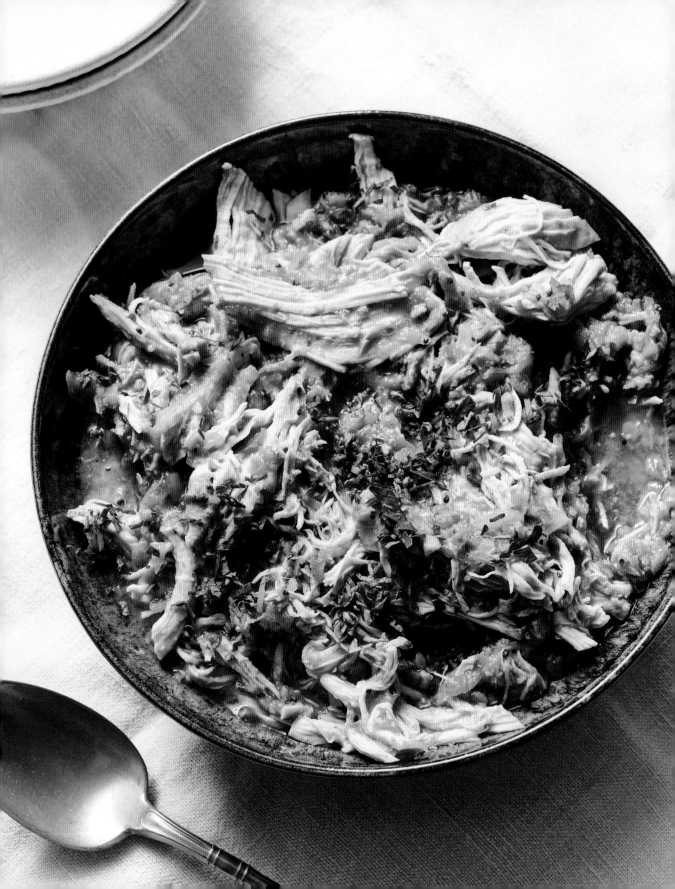

MUSTARD MAPLE CHICKEN
WITH SWEET POTATO

The sweet flavours and tender chicken make this a popular family-friendly dish. You can simply serve it with steamed green vegetables, such as broccoli, asparagus or green beans, or cook some rice to make it into a more substantial meal.

PREP TIME: 10 MINUTES

COOK TIME: 2–3 HOURS (HIGH) OR 4–6 HOURS (LOW)

2 carrots (total weight about 200g / 7oz), grated

1 onion, finely chopped

3 sweet potatoes (total weight 350–400g / 12–14oz), peeled and cut into 1cm/½ inch sized cubes

4 skinless chicken breasts

2 tablespoons pure maple syrup

1 tablespoon apple cider vinegar

2 teaspoons wholegrain mustard

2 garlic cloves, crushed

1 teaspoon dried sage

1 teaspoon salt

½ teaspoon pepper

100ml (3½fl oz) hot water

handful of parsley leaves, finely chopped, to serve

1. Put the carrots, onion, sweet potatoes and chicken breasts into the slow-cooker pot.

2. In a small bowl, mix up the maple syrup, vinegar, mustard, garlic, sage, salt, pepper and the hot water, then pour over all the ingredients in the slow-cooker bowl.

3. Give everything a stir to make sure the sauce has dispersed, place the lid on, and cook on high for 2–3 hours, or on low for 4–6 hours. After the cooking time, the chicken should be tender and easy to pull apart with 2 forks into the sauce.

4. Pull the chicken and mix it through the sauce before serving scattered with chopped parsley.

NOTE To cook this in a regular oven, preheat the oven to 220°C/200°C fan (425°F), Gas Mark 7. Place all the ingredients into a casserole dish and cover with a lid, or into a baking dish and cover with foil, and bake for 35–45 minutes until the chicken is tender and easy to pull apart.

PER SERVING: Calories 378 | Fat 3.4g | Sat Fat 0.8g | Carbs 47g | Sugars 23g | Fibre 6.2g | Protein 37g | Salt 1.9g

CREAMY CHINESE FIVE SPICE CHICKEN CURRY

A creamy curry, packed with the easy-to-access flavours of five spice and curry powder, this makes a great fakeaway with the most minimal input. Serve it with rice or noodles. I also sometimes cook some frozen peas and add them to the dish, although you could serve it with stir-fried vegetables.

PREP TIME: 5 MINUTES
**COOK TIME: 4–5 HOURS (HIGH)
OR 6–7 HOURS (LOW)**

1 onion, finely chopped
3 garlic cloves, crushed
1 tablespoon tomato purée
400ml (14fl oz) can of light
   coconut milk
1 tablespoon mild curry powder
1 tablespoon ground turmeric
1 teaspoon Chinese five spice
1 teaspoon salt
½ teaspoon chilli flakes
3 skinless chicken breasts
3 spring onions, sliced, to serve

1. Put the onion, garlic, tomato purée, coconut milk, curry powder, turmeric, Chinese five spice, salt and chilli flakes into the slow-cooker pot and mix everything together.
2. Submerge the chicken breasts in the sauce and cook on high for 4–5 hours, or on low for 6–7 hours. When it's done the chicken should be tender and easy to pull apart.
3. Shred the chicken into the sauce with 2 forks to thicken everything up and soak those flavours into the chicken.
4. Serve scattered with the spring onions.

NOTE You can add some extra vegetables to cook in the sauce if you like. Add carrot sticks or sliced peppers along with the chicken, or try peas or mushrooms added 30 minutes before the end of cooking time.

To cook this in a regular oven, preheat the oven to 210°C/190°C fan (410°F), Gas Mark 6½. Put all the ingredients in a casserole dish, cover with the lid and cook for 55 minutes until the chicken is tender and easy to pull apart.

PER SERVING: Calories 222 | Fat 9.1g | Sat Fat 6.7g | Carbs 6.6g | Sugars 4.1g | Fibre 2g | Protein 27g | Salt 1.6g

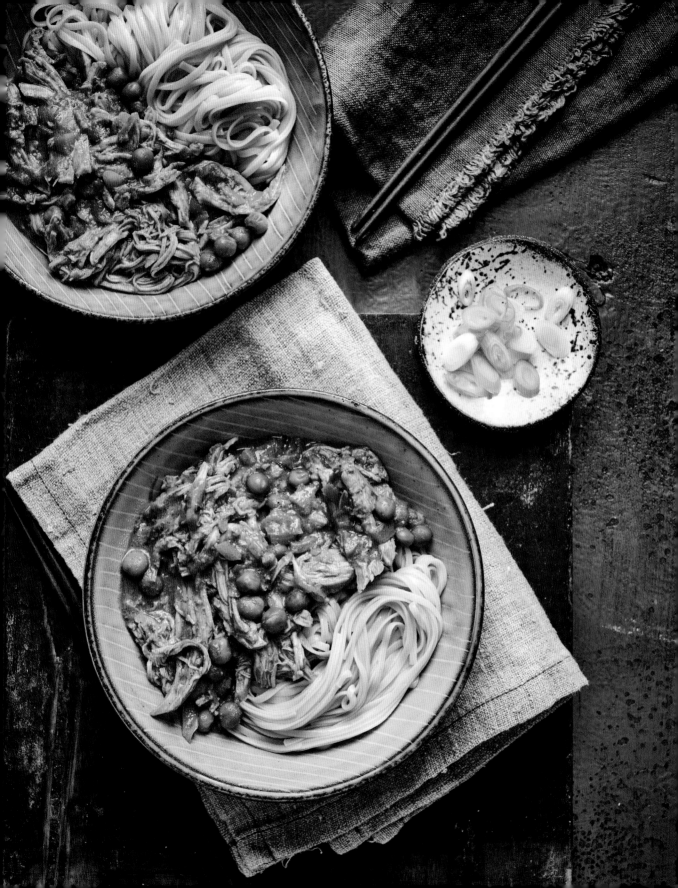

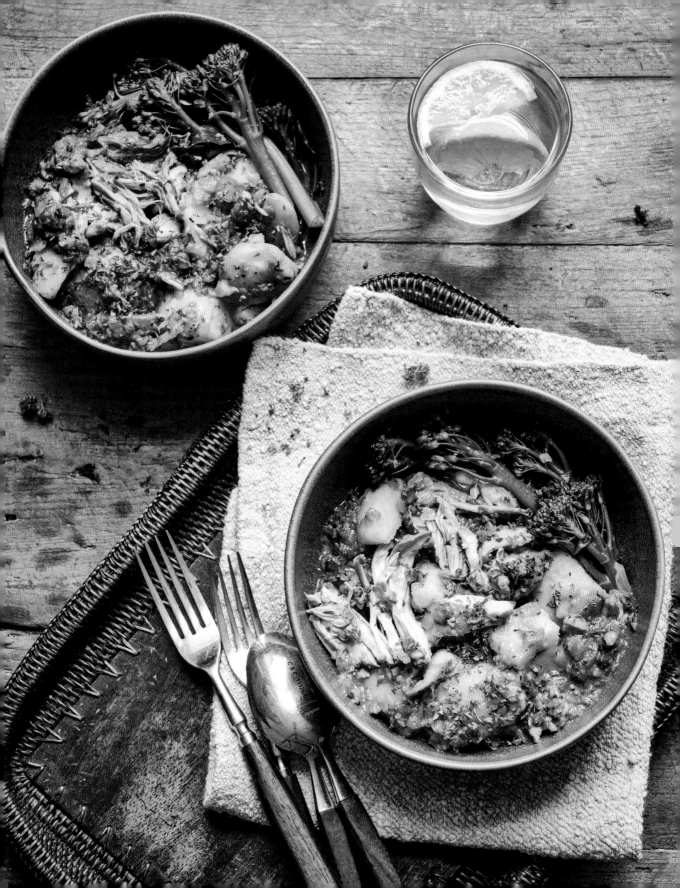

SERVES 4

COSY CHICKEN LEMON & POTATO CASSEROLE

This is one of my girls' favourite meals, which is great for me as it's quick to prep and the sort of meal I will throw together before we go to the beach on a cold day; it's the perfect food to come home to and warm up (which is why my daughter calls it 'cosy casserole'). The chicken is tender, the potatoes soft and everything is gently flavoured with herbs and lemon. I'll serve this up with whatever green vegetables I have, usually broccoli, green beans or asparagus, or frozen peas.

PREP TIME: 10 MINUTES

COOK TIME: 4–5 HOURS (HIGH) OR 7–8 HOURS (LOW)

1 onion, finely chopped (see note)
6 skinless chicken thigh fillets, excess fat trimmed away
800g (1lb 12oz) potatoes, such as Maris Piper, quartered
3 garlic cloves, crushed
500ml (18fl oz) hot chicken stock
1 teaspoon dried oregano
1 teaspoon dried basil
1 teaspoon dried rosemary
finely grated zest and juice of 1 lemon
salt and pepper, to taste
handful of parsley leaves, finely chopped, to serve

1. Place the onion in a small bowl and microwave for 3 minutes, stirring halfway through.
2. Put all the ingredients, including the onion, into the slow-cooker, give everything a stir, and cook on high for 4–5 hours, or on low for 7–8 hours. When it's done the chicken should be tender and easy to pull apart.
3. Serve scattered with parsley.

NOTE Raw onions can be added to a slow-cooker for most dishes, but you will sometimes find that it slightly alters the final flavour of the dish, which is why many recipes recommend frying them first. The downside of this is that it adds precious minutes to the prep time and also gets another pan dirty. My solution in a dish like this, where the flavours are quite subtle and I don't want the onions adding too much sharpness, is to cook them first in the microwave for a few minutes. This will soften and sweeten them but can also be done in the time that it takes to put all the other ingredients into the slow-cooker.

To cook this in a regular oven, preheat the oven to 180°C/160°C fan (350°F), Gas Mark 4. Put all the ingredients in a casserole dish, cover with the lid and cook for 1 hour 20 minutes.

PER SERVING: Calories 369 | Fat 9.5g | Sat Fat 2.6g | Carbs 40g | Sugars 5.2g | Fibre 5.5g | Protein 27g | Salt 2.3g

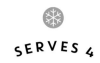

CREAMY PEANUT PULLED PORK

This dish has all the key satay flavours in a creamy sauce. Slow cooking the pork means it's tender and easy to shred. I love this served with rice and crunchy veg such as baby corn and green beans. Garlic and ginger pastes save on preparation time, but you could substitute these for crushed garlic cloves and finely grated fresh root ginger.

PREP TIME: 5 MINUTES
COOK TIME: 4–6 HOURS (HIGH) OR 6–8 HOURS (LOW)

1 pork tenderloin (about 500g / 1lb 2oz)

3 sweet peppers (red, yellow or orange), deseeded and chopped

2 tablespoons peanut butter

2 tablespoons dark soy sauce

1 tablespoon rice wine

2 teaspoons garlic paste

2 teaspoons ginger paste

1 teaspoon chilli flakes

400ml (14fl oz) can of light coconut milk

1 tablespoon cornflour

TO SERVE
lime wedges
coriander leaves

1. Put the pork and peppers into the slow-cooker.
2. In a bowl, mix up the peanut butter, soy sauce, rice wine, garlic, ginger and chilli flakes with the coconut milk so that all of the ingredients have dispersed. Mix the cornflour with a little water in a small cup until you have a smooth liquid, then stir this in, too.
3. Add the coconut milk mixture to the slow-cooker, pouring it all over the pork and peppers.
4. Cook on high for 4–6 hours, or on low for 6–8 hours. At the end of the cooking time the pork should be easy to shred into the sauce with 2 forks.
5. Serve scattered with coriander and with lime wedges on the side.

NOTE You can adjust this to your taste: if you want it more peanutty, add a couple more tablespoons of peanut butter (the amount I use here adds flavour but without increasing the calorie count too much). You could add sweet potato or butternut squash chunks instead of – or as well as – the peppers. You can leave out the chilli, or add more. If you are serving more people, you can add an extra pork tenderloin.

To cook this in a regular oven, preheat the oven to 200°C/180°C fan (400°F), Gas Mark 6. Put all the ingredients in a casserole dish, cover with the lid and cook for 2 hours.

PER SERVING: Calories 341 | Fat 16g | Sat Fat 8.9g | Carbs 15g | Sugars 8.9g | Fibre 3.5g | Protein 32g | Salt 1.8g

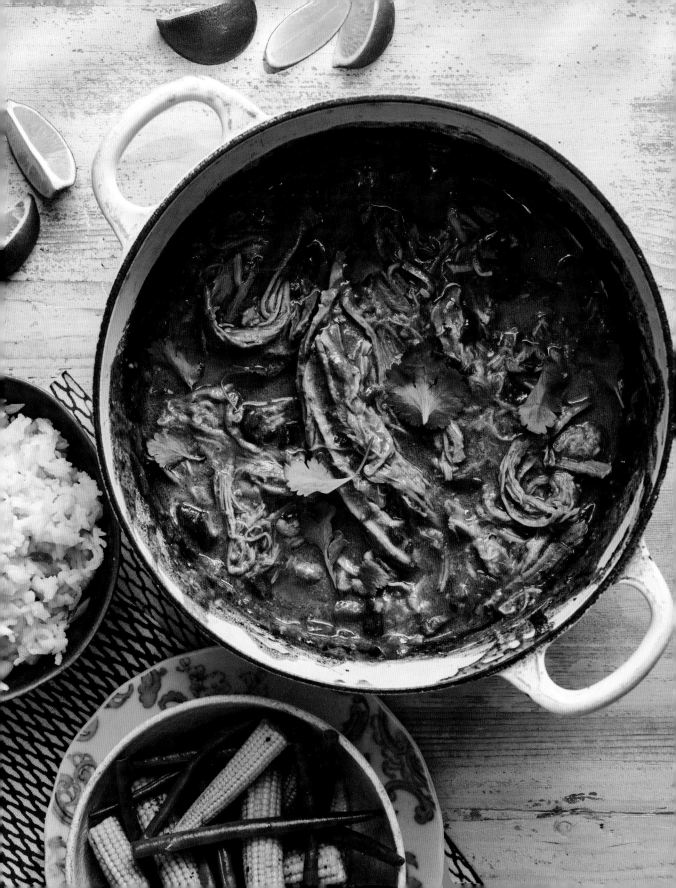

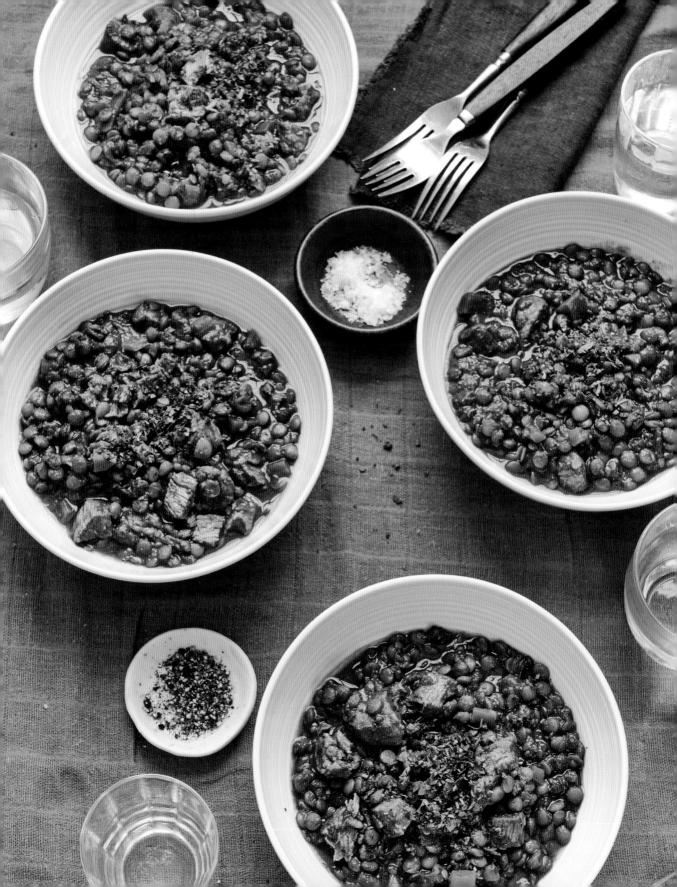

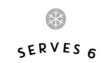

UNCLE PAUL'S RICH SPICED LAMB & LENTILS

My husband's Uncle Paul once made us a really delicious slow-cooker lamb shank and lentil curry, which I have always remembered as being so tasty and satisfying to eat. Lamb shanks aren't always easy to get hold of, so I have substituted these with simple diced lamb leg, which still works brilliantly with the rich, tomatoey lentil sauce. One of the joys of this one-pot is that there is only the smallest amount of chopping involved: all the flavour comes from a simple mix of spices, tomatoes and the lamb itself.

PREP TIME: 5 MINUTES

COOK TIME: 4–5 HOURS (HIGH) OR 8–10 HOURS (LOW)

600g (1lb 5oz) diced lamb leg
300g (10½oz) dry green lentils
20g (¾oz) dry red lentils
400g (14oz) can of chopped tomatoes
2 carrots, finely chopped
750ml (1 pint 5fl oz) lamb stock
1 cinnamon stick
handful of parsley leaves, finely chopped, to serve

FOR THE SPICE PASTE
4 tablespoons tomato purée
1 tablespoon garam masala
1 teaspoon ground turmeric
1 teaspoon cayenne pepper
1 teaspoon garlic granules
1 teaspoon onion granules
1 teaspoon salt

1. In a small bowl, mix together all the ingredients for the spice paste.
2. Pop the diced lamb into the slow-cooker pot and stir in the spice paste until the lamb is fully coated.
3. Add the lentils, tomatoes, carrots and stock and give everything a stir. Add the cinnamon stick to the pot.
4. Cook on high for 4–5 hours, or on low for 8–10 hours. Serve scattered with parsley.

NOTE To cook this in a regular oven, preheat the oven to 170°C/150°C fan (340°F), Gas Mark 3½. Put all the ingredients in a casserole dish, cover with the lid and cook for 1½ hours.

PER SERVING: Calories 412 | Fat 11g | Sat Fat 4g | Carbs 33g | Sugars 8g | Fibre 7.6g | Protein 41g | Salt 1.4g

SERVES 8

KOREAN-STYLE GOCHUJANG BEEF BRISKET

This is not a traditional Korean dish, but Korean gochujang is the key flavour to make a really delicious sauce for beef brisket, which, after slow cooking, will shred perfectly. I served it up at a birthday dinner with jasmine rice, a quick red cabbage and carrot 'slaw and some shredded Little Gem lettuce. To speed up the prep time even more, you can use pre-chopped, frozen butternut squash and onion.

PREP TIME: 15 MINUTES

COOK TIME: 4–5 HOURS (HIGH) OR 6–8 HOURS (LOW)

2 large onions, finely sliced

1 tablespoon cornflour

350g (12oz) butternut squash, cut into about 1cm (½ inch) pieces

2 large carrots, cut into matchsticks

1 eating apple, peeled, cored and chopped

800g–1kg (1lb 12oz–2lb 4oz) rolled beef brisket

4 garlic cloves, crushed

5cm (2 inch) piece of fresh root ginger, peeled and finely grated

2 tablespoons gochujang paste

3 tablespoons light soy sauce

2 tablespoons apple cider vinegar

1 tablespoon honey

150ml (¼ pint) apple juice

spring onions, sliced, to serve

1. Put the onions and cornflour into the slow-cooker and stir together. Add the squash, carrot sticks and apple.

2. Remove any butcher's string from the beef and place it into the slow-cooker.

3. In a bowl, mix together the garlic, ginger, gochujang, soy sauce, vinegar, honey and apple juice to make a sauce, then pour this all over the beef and vegetables.

4. Cook on high for 4–5 hours, or on low for 6–8 hours.

5. When cooked, the beef should be tender and easy to shred. Shred it with 2 forks and stir it into the juices and vegetables before serving, scattered with spring onions.

NOTE To cook this in a regular oven, preheat the oven to 170°C/150°C fan (340°F), Gas Mark 3½. Put all the ingredients in a casserole dish, cover with the lid and cook for 4 hours.

PER SERVING: Calories 325 | Fat 12g | Sat Fat 4.3g | Carbs 21g | Sugars 14g | Fibre 3.7g | Protein 30g | Salt 1.4g

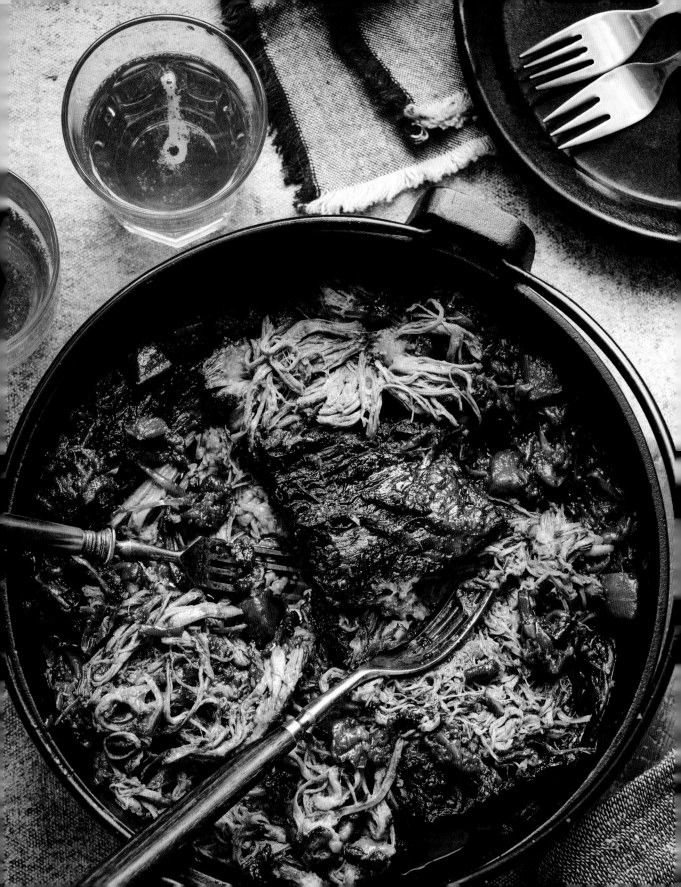

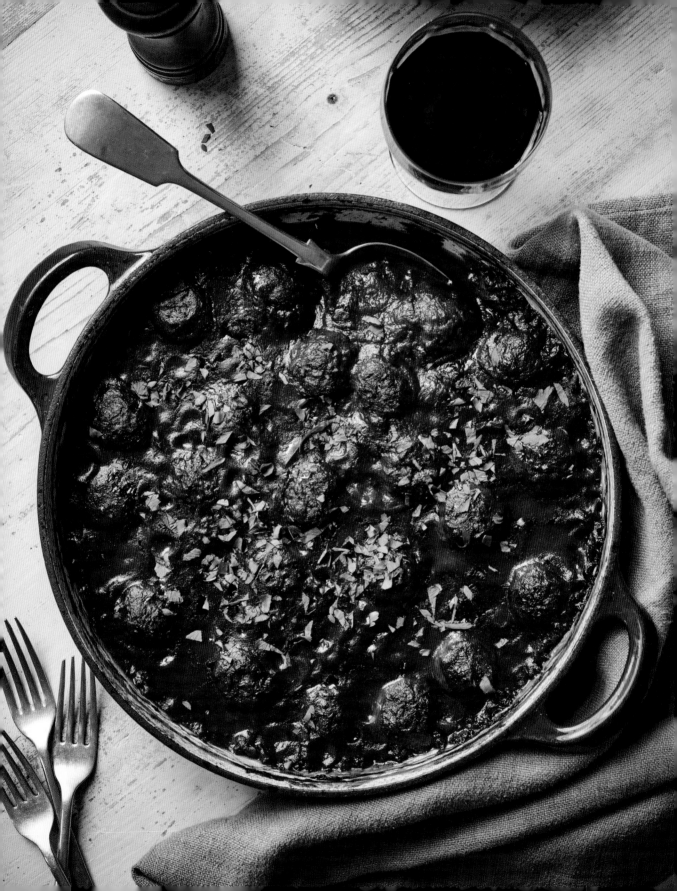

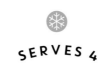

MARRY-ME MEATBALLS

Meatballs were the first meal I ever made for my husband. I used a whole Scotch bonnet chilli and they were so, so hot that they were almost inedible. I still love making meatballs, but have toned down the spice! These meatballs are a winner because you just make them up and dunk them into the sauce, leaving the slow-cooker to develop a flavoursome sauce and tender meatballs. Serve these with your favourite pasta, or for a lighter option, courgetti.

PREP TIME: 20 MINUTES

COOK TIME: 4–5 HOURS (HIGH) OR 6–8 HOURS (LOW)

500g (1lb 2oz) lean minced beef (5 per cent fat)
1 teaspoon Italian-style mixed dried herbs
¼ teaspoon fennel seeds
1 large carrot, grated
handful of parsley or basil leaves, finely chopped, to serve

FOR THE SAUCE
400g (14oz) can of chopped tomatoes
500g (1lb 2oz) tomato passata
2 tablespoons tomato purée
150ml (¼ pint) red wine
1 onion, finely chopped
4 garlic cloves, crushed
1 red pepper, deseeded and chopped
1 beef stock cube, crumbled
1 tablespoon Italian-style mixed dried herbs
1 teaspoon sugar
½ teaspoon salt
½ teaspoon pepper

1. Put all the sauce ingredients in the slow-cooker bowl and mix them together thoroughly.
2. In a large bowl, mix together the meatball ingredients and use your hands to form walnut-sized meatballs (I make about 22, though you can make smaller ones if you prefer). Gently submerge the meatballs into the sauce as you make them.
3. Cook on high for 4–5 hours, or on low for 6–8 hours. Serve scattered with chopped parsley or basil.

NOTE If you are really short on time, you could consider using lean ready-made meatballs from the supermarket. If you have kids who won't eat sauce containing chunky veg, then, once this is cooked, fish out the meatballs and just use a stick blender to blitz the rest into a nice smooth sauce which will work for the fussiest of eaters!

To cook this in a regular oven, preheat the oven to 180°C/160°C fan (350°F), Gas Mark 4. Put all the ingredients in a casserole dish, cover with the lid and cook for 1 hour.

PER SERVING: Calories 313 | Fat 5.8g | Sat Fat 2.5g | Carbs 21g | Sugars 19g | Fibre 7.2g | Protein 32g | Salt 2g

BEEF, BUTTERNUT & SPINACH STEW

A great, warming comfort dish, full of goodness and the subtle flavours of cinnamon and paprika. Prunes might seem like an unlikely addition, but they add a lovely sweetness and extra depth of flavour – I just don't tell anyone they are in there! Serve with mashed potato and green veg, or with any of my Couscous recipes (see pages 94–99).

PREP TIME: 15 MINUTES

COOK TIME: 4–5 HOURS (HIGH) OR 6–8 HOURS (LOW)

600g (1lb 5oz) lean diced beef
1 tablespoon cornflour
650g (1lb 7oz) butternut squash, cut into cubes (you can use frozen)
1 red onion, finely chopped
4 garlic cloves, crushed
80g (2¾oz) pitted prunes, finely chopped
1 tablespoon thyme leaves
large handful of parsley leaves, finely chopped
400g (14oz) can of chopped tomatoes
2 tablespoons tomato purée
500ml (18fl oz) hot beef stock
1 tablespoon apple cider vinegar
1 cinnamon stick
1 bay leaf
1 teaspoon sweet paprika
½ teaspoon ground cumin
4 large handfuls of baby spinach
salt and pepper, to taste

1. Tip the beef into the slow-cooker and stir in the cornflour.
2. Add all the rest of the ingredients apart from the spinach, season with salt and pepper and give it all a good mix.
3. Set it cooking for 4–5 hours on high, or 6–8 hours on low.
4. Once the cooking time is up, stir in the spinach leaves until they have wilted, then serve.

NOTE To cook this in a regular oven, preheat the oven to 180°C/160°C fan (350°F), Gas Mark 4. Put all the ingredients in a casserole dish, cover with the lid and cook for 1½ hours.

PER SERVING: Calories 266 | Fat 6.1g | Sat Fat 2.1g | Carbs 24g | Sugars 15g | Fibre 4.8g | Protein 26g | Salt 0.81g

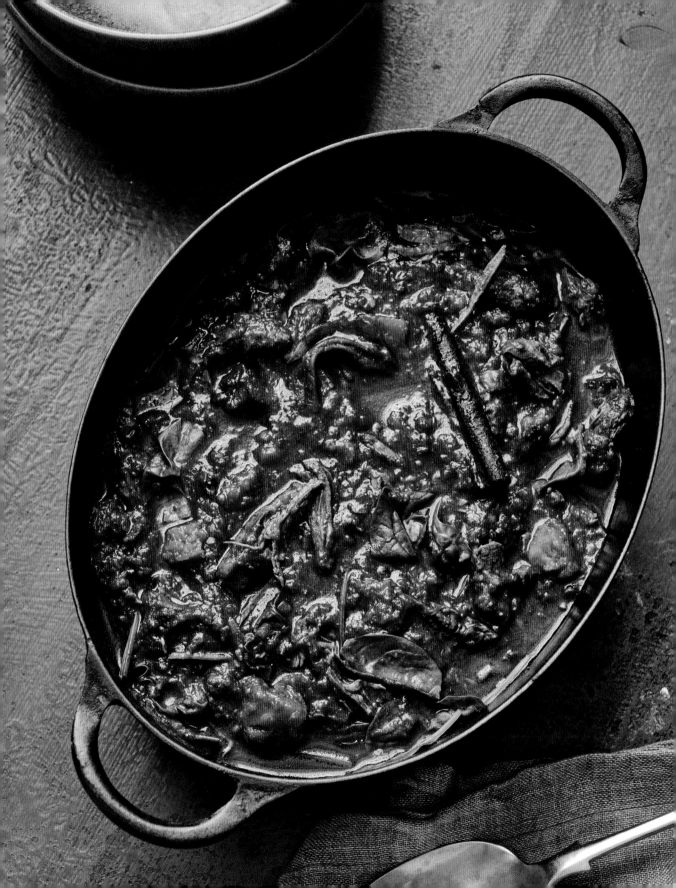

CHAPTER 7

SNACKS & SIDES

CREAMY LEMON DIP

It's always useful to have some quick dip ideas up your sleeve, because they can make a great snack, or give you a quick and easy nibble to serve up when friends or family pop over. Butter beans are great for dips as they have soft skins, so blend super-smoothly. With the added luxury of cream cheese, this is a really indulgent-tasting savoury dip that goes perfectly with wraps or pittas cut into slices and oven baked for a few minutes until crisp, crudités, or even as an alternative to butter in a sandwich: try it spread over wholemeal or seeded bread with chicken or smoked salmon.

PREP TIME: 5 MINUTES

COOK TIME: NONE

400g (14oz) can of butter beans, drained and rinsed

finely grated zest and juice of 1 lemon

3 tablespoons fat-free Greek yogurt

2 tablespoons reduced-fat cream cheese

1 small garlic clove

½ teaspoon dried thyme

½ teaspoon salt

1. Place all the ingredients into a mini chopper and blend until you have a smooth and creamy dip.

NOTE This base makes a great starting point for all sorts of flavoured dips. Try omitting the lemon and thyme and customizing with your favourite spices or spice blends: smoked paprika, za'atar, chipotle chilli flakes or Italian-style mixed dried herbs all work well. If you aren't using the lemon juice, you might just need to add a little extra Greek yogurt to make it the perfect smooth consistency.

PER SERVING: Calories 64 | Fat 0.9g | Sat Fat 0.4g | Carbs 6.6g | Sugars 2.2g | Fibre 1.9g | Protein 5.5g | Salt 0.47g

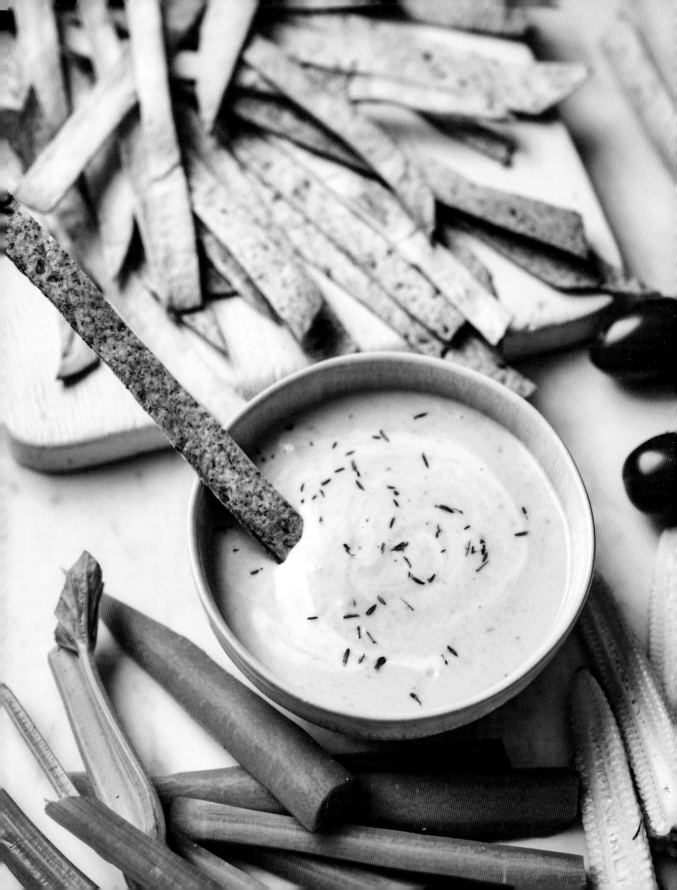

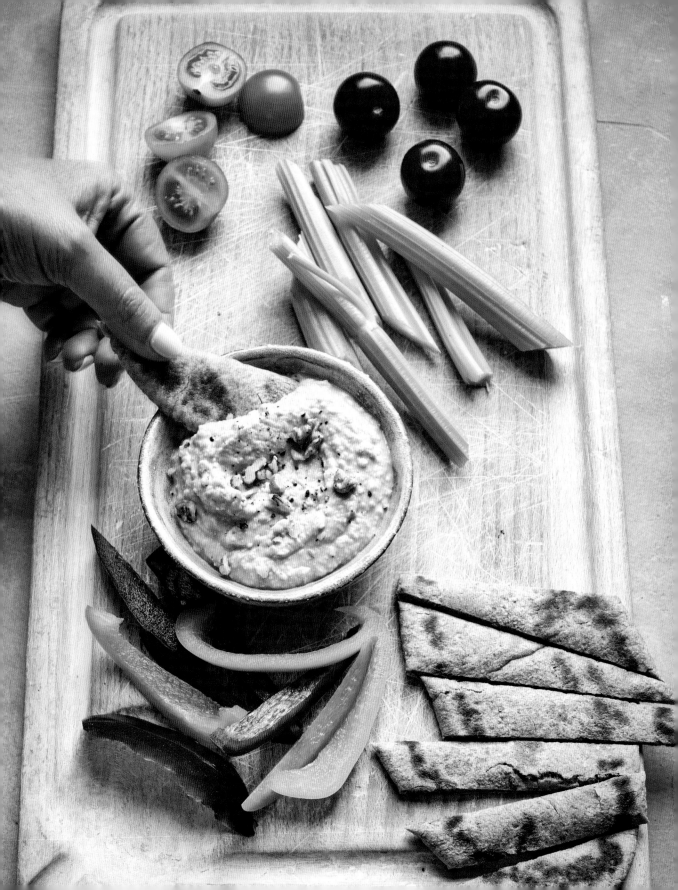

TOASTED WALNUT HUMMUS

Homemade hummus is such a simple way to boost meals and snacks. A handful of lightly toasted walnuts adds earthy, rich flavour to a simple hummus in this recipe. This will pair well with my Beetroot, Kale & Chilli Falafel, or my Baked Lamb Kofta with Mint & Yogurt Sauce in Pitta (see pages 39 and 125), or simply serve with crudités and toasted pitta.

PREP TIME: 5 MINUTES

COOK TIME: 5 MINUTES

25g (1oz) walnut halves

400g (14oz) can of chickpeas, drained and rinsed

2 garlic cloves

juice of ½ lemon

½ teaspoon salt

3 tablespoons fat-free Greek yogurt

1. In a small frying pan, dry-fry the walnut halves for 5 minutes, stirring all the time to prevent any parts catching and burning. The aim is to bring out the natural sweetness of toasted walnuts without any bitter burned bits.

2. Place the walnuts, chickpeas, garlic, lemon juice, salt and yogurt into a food processor and blend until smooth.

3. Serve immediately or store in an airtight container in the refrigerator for up to 5 days.

NOTE Some other tasty ways to add different flavours to this hummus are a roasted red pepper in brine from a jar, or smoked paprika, a fresh chilli, or even pre-roasted carrots: just blend the extra ingredient in with everything else.

PER SERVING: Calories 137 | Fat 5.7g | Sat Fat 0.5g | Carbs 11g | Sugars 1.8g | Fibre 3.3g | Protein 8.1g | Salt 0.65

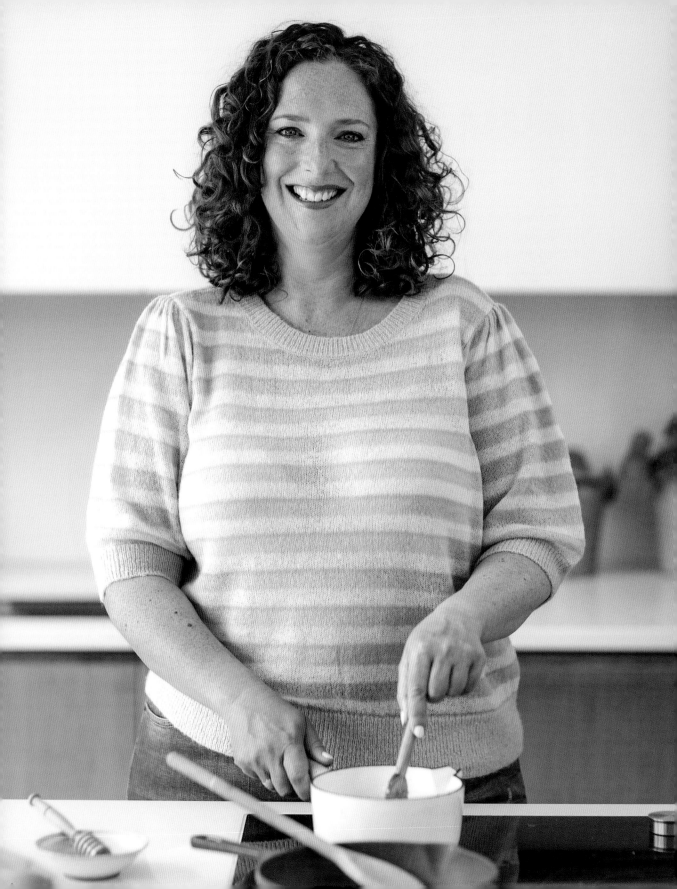

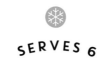

GA'S SMOKED MACKEREL & HORSERADISH PÂTÉ

My friend Hannah mentioned that her mother-in-law makes an amazing pâté with smoked mackerel, horseradish and cottage cheese and it sounded right up my street, so I thought I would have a go! I've used quark (a fat-free cheese with the consistency of thick yogurt) instead of cottage cheese, because I find it easier to get hold of. You can serve this as a sandwich filling, a jacket potato topping, a dip for crudités, or spread over crackers (try my Oat, Chickpea & Herb Crackers, see page 196). Recipe pictured on page 196.

PREP TIME: 5 MINUTES
COOK TIME: NONE

300g (10½oz) smoked mackerel fillets, skinned
4 tablespoons quark, plus extra if needed
finely grated zest and juice of ½ lemon
1 tablespoon horseradish sauce (see note)
salt and pepper, to taste

TO SERVE (OPTIONAL)
sliced spring onions
cress

1. If you want a smooth pâté, roughly tear the skinned mackerel fillets into the bowl of a food processor, then add the quark, lemon juice, horseradish and some salt and pepper. Blend until you have a smooth pâté. If it's looking a little dry, you can add some more quark to keep it smooth.

2. If you want a more textured pâté, then simply flake the smoked mackerel into pieces, then stir in the quark, lemon juice, horseradish and salt and pepper to taste.

3. Scatter with the lemon zest and add spring onions or snipped cress, if you like. This will keep for up to 3 days in a sealed container in the refrigerator (but don't scatter anything on top until ready to serve). If you aren't eating it immediately, you may just need to give it a little stir before serving, as it can separate a bit as it sits.

NOTE The power of horseradish sauce varies hugely; some are so peppery that just a tiny taste will almost have you sneezing, whereas others are much milder. I use 1 tablespoon for this recipe, but there is always room for more if you want a stronger flavour! Just adjust it to your own taste.

PER SERVING: Calories 166 | Fat 11g | Sat Fat 2.5g | Carbs 1.9g | Sugars 1.8g | Fibre 0.5g | Protein 1.3g | Salt 1.3g

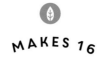

OAT, CHICKPEA & HERB CRACKERS

This is a really simple method to make healthy crackers that are just perfect for easy lunches or snacks. I have used a herbes de Provence mix in these, but you can customize them with your favourite herbs or spices: I love a chilli version and also just plain rosemary. Try serving them with my Smoked Mackerel & Horseradish Paté (see page 195).

PREP TIME: 10 MINUTES
COOK TIME: 15 MINUTES

400g (14oz) can of chickpeas, drained and rinsed
80g (2¾oz) oats
1 egg white
2 teaspoons herbes de Provence
1/2 teaspoon coarse salt

1. Preheat the oven to 220°C/200°C fan (425°F), Gas Mark 7. Line a large baking tray with nonstick baking paper.
2. Put the chickpeas into a food processor and whizz them to a crumb-like consistency. Add the oats and whizz again until very finely chopped.
3. Add the egg white, herbs and salt and process until the mixture starts to clump and form a dough-like ball. Remove the dough from the food processor and shape into a ball.
4. Place the dough between 2 sheets of nonstick baking paper, press down to flatten slightly, then use a rolling pin to roll it out into a rectangle, 3–4mm (⅛ inch) thick.
5. Use a sharp knife to cut away and neaten the edges, then cut the dough into crackers about 5 × 3cm (2 × 1¼ inches) each. Roll out the remaining dough from the edges and repeat, or just cut these into more rustic shapes!
6. Prick each cracker a couple of times with a fork, transfer carefully to the prepared tray and bake for 15 minutes until crisp around the edges and golden in colour.

NOTE These come out of the oven with a lovely crunch, but they can soften up once stored. You can always give them a quick blast in a hot oven to crisp them up again, and allow them to fully cool before you seal them into a container (where they will last for 4–5 days).

PER CRACKER: Calories 39 | Fat 0.8g | Sat Fat 0.1g | Carbs 5.4g | Sugars 0g | Fibre 1.1g | Protein 1.9g | Salt 0.16g

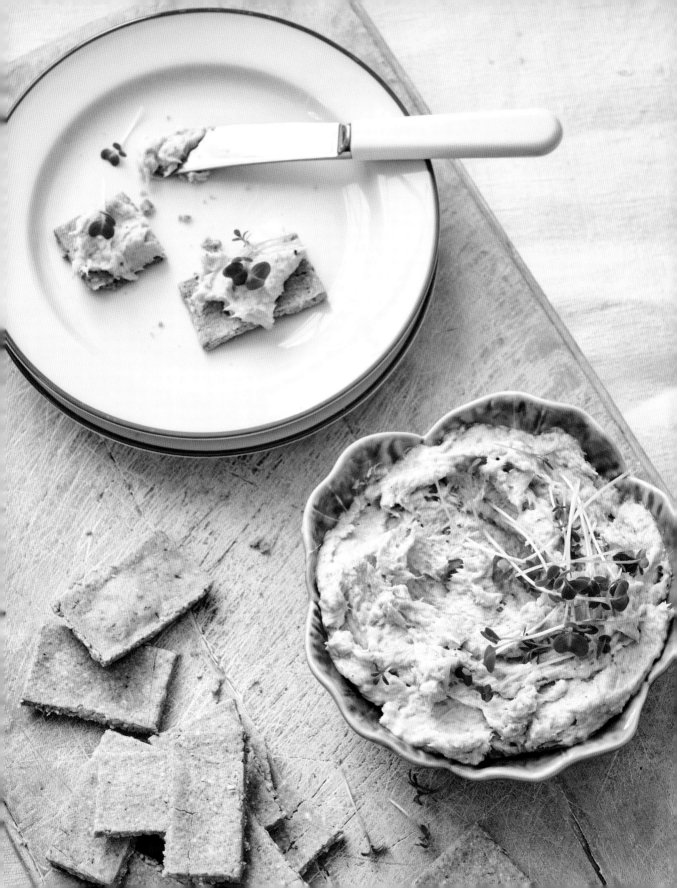

CRISP GREEN SALAD
WITH KOREAN-STYLE DRESSING

A refreshingly crispy salad with a hot and sweet dressing.

PREP TIME: 5 MINUTES
COOK TIME: 2 MINUTES

2 Sweet Gem or 4 Little Gem
   lettuces
½ cucumber
2 eating apples
juice of ½ lemon

FOR THE DRESSING
1 tablespoon sesame seeds
½ tablespoon gochujang paste
1 tablespoon rice vinegar
1 tablespoon light soy sauce
1 garlic clove, crushed
1 teaspoon honey

1. Trim the stalks from the lettuces then cut them into strips. Halve the cucumber lengthways and finely slice it.
2. Peel and core the apples, then quarter them and finely slice. As soon as the apples are sliced, mix them with the lemon juice in a small bowl so they don't turn brown.
3. Dry-fry the sesame seeds in a small frying pan for 2 minutes until they are lightly toasted.
4. In a small bowl, mix together all the dressing ingredients, including the toasted sesame seeds, ensuring you have a smooth dressing with no lumps.
5. Put the lettuce, cucumber and apples into a bowl and toss through the dressing. Serve.

NOTE Add any extra crunchy veg that you fancy to this, such as radishes, sweet peppers, bean sprouts or carrots cut into matchsticks.

PER SERVING: Calories 93 | Fat 2.5g | Sat Fat 0.4g | Carbs 13g | Sugars 11g | Fibre 2.4g | Protein 2.6g | Salt 0.62g

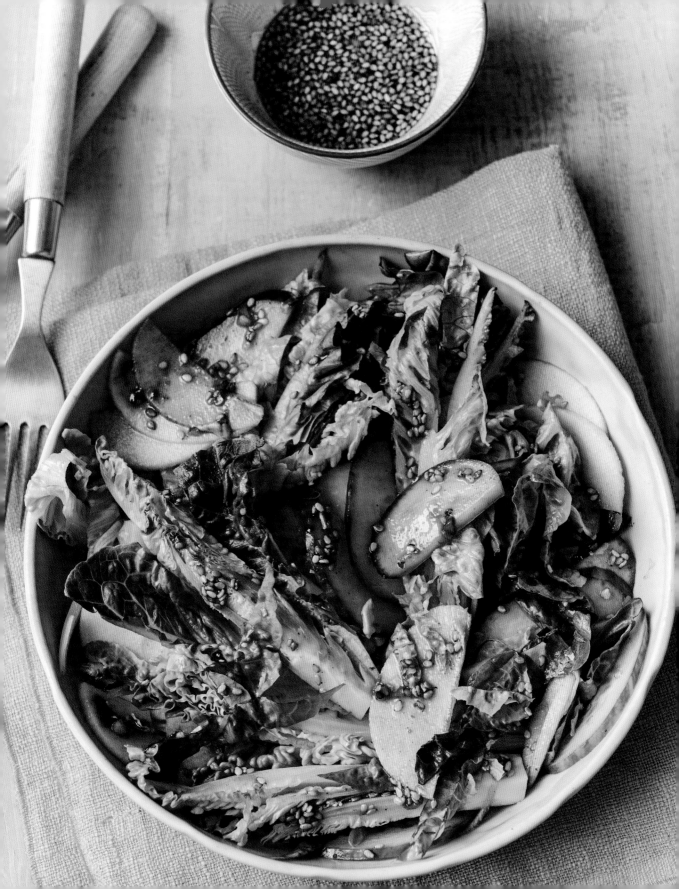

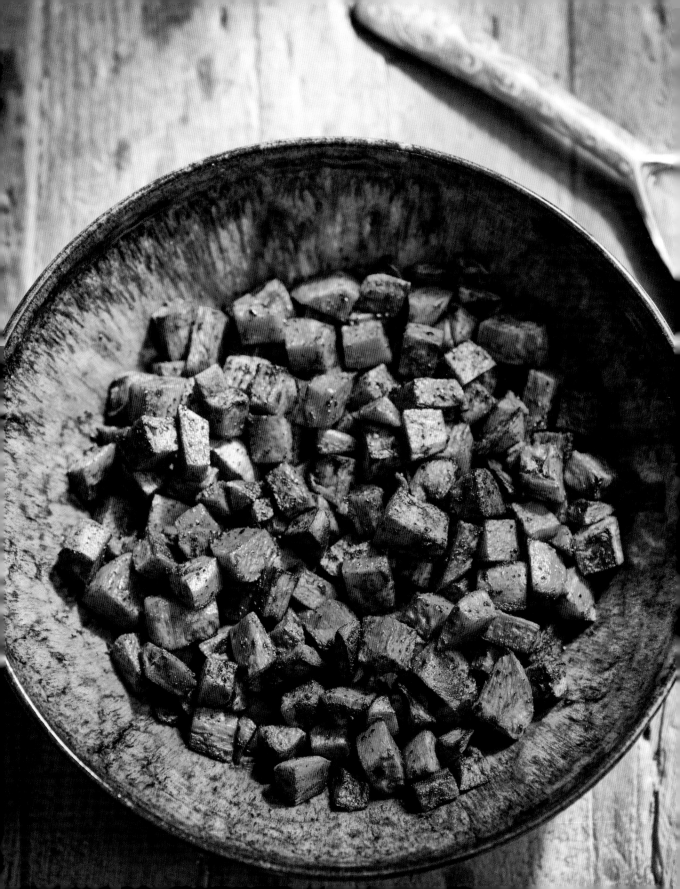

SUMAC-ROASTED SWEET POTATOES

The sweet and citrussy flavour of sumac on sweet potatoes is just delicious, plus they look so pretty once roasted. These work really well with salads, meats, fish, alongside curries . . . they are just easy and versatile. I usually use low-calorie cooking spray rather than oil when I am baking potatoes or sweet potatoes, as it gives great coverage and helps to crisp them up without the need for lots of oil.

PREP TIME: 5 MINUTES

COOK TIME: 20 MINUTES

3–4 sweet potatoes, peeled and cut into about 2cm (¾ inch) chunks

salt and pepper, to taste

1 tablespoon sumac

1 teaspoon coarse salt

½ teaspoon smoked paprika

low-calorie cooking spray

1. Preheat the oven to 220°C/200°C fan (425°F), Gas Mark 7. Line a large baking tray with nonstick baking paper.
2. Place the sweet potato cubes in a large bowl, add the sumac, salt and smoked paprika and toss everything together until the potatoes are evenly covered.
3. Spray the potatoes generously with low-calorie cooking spray and toss again.
4. Spread out on the prepared tray in a single layer.
5. Place in the oven and bake for 20 minutes, by which time they should be golden on the outside and fudgy and soft within.

NOTE These are also great with a spicy element such as cayenne or chilli added. There is no need to peel sweet potatoes if the skins are in good condition, they are great either way.

PER SERVING: Calories 179 | Fat 1.5g | Sat Fat 0.4g | Carbs 37g | Sugars 9.9g | Fibre 5.5g | Protein 2.3g | Salt 1.5g

CHERMOULA

Chermoula is a condiment that resembles a North African-flavoured pesto, typically with lemon, garlic, coriander, parsley and a mixture of spices. I have spotted this more often available as a paste in British supermarkets, and, as with most things, a freshly made version tastes much better. I have kept my recipe very simple, with no need to toast spices or source rare ingredients. You can use this in so many ways, because it makes a brilliant basis for a quick meal that is bursting with flavour (see note). Although traditionally a mortar and pestle would be used, I use a mini chopper or food processor to make it quickly and easily.

PREP TIME: 5 MINUTES
COOK TIME: NONE

20g (¾oz) bunch of coriander
10g (¼oz) bunch of parsley
2cm (¾ inch) piece of fresh
   root ginger, peeled and
   roughly chopped
2 garlic cloves
1 teaspoon ground cumin
1 teaspoon ground coriander
1 teaspoon sweet paprika
¼ teaspoon chilli flakes
¼ teaspoon salt
finely grated zest and juice of
   1 lemon
1 teaspoon olive oil

1. Place all the ingredients into a mini chopper or small food processor bowl and pulse together until you have a paste.

NOTE Chermoula is a fabulous all-rounder. Use it to marinate meat or fish, or baste meat or fish during and after cooking. It is a great near-instant sauce, or can be spooned into soup or stew for extra flavour. Or try stirring it through couscous, or stir-fried or roasted vegetables, for a zing of flavour.

PER SERVING: Calories 30 | Fat 1.5g | Sat Fat 0.2g | Carbs 1.8g | Sugars 1.2g | Fibre 0.7g | Protein 0.8g | Salt 0.33g

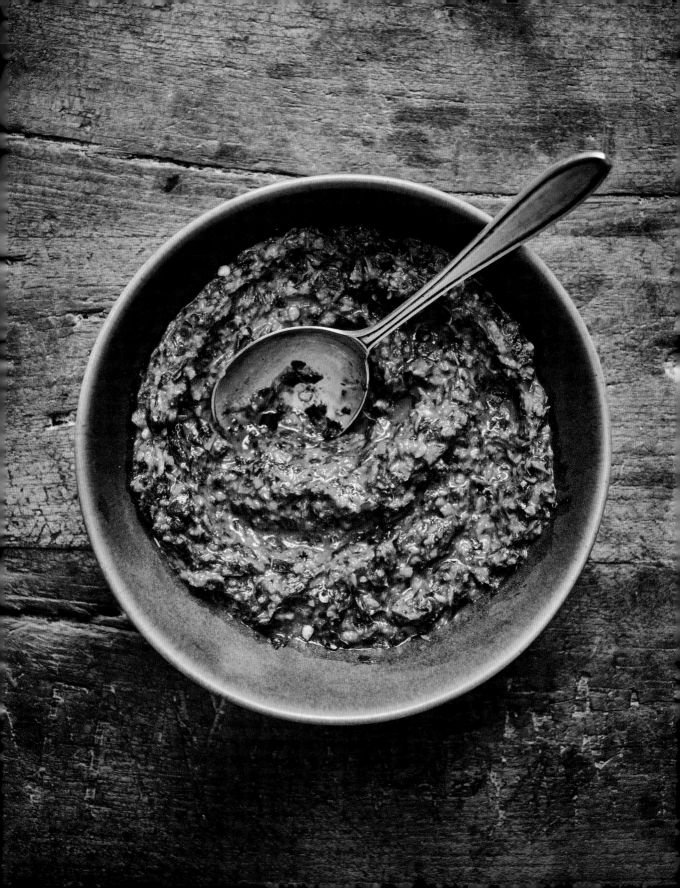

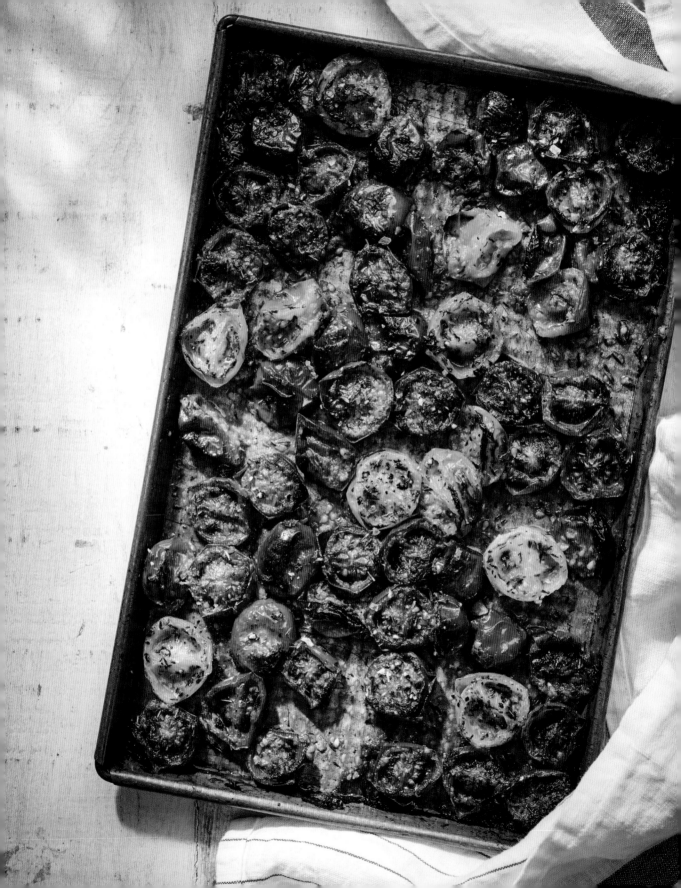

FLAVOUR-BOMB ROAST CHERRY TOMATOES

I tend to make these when I have cherry tomatoes in the refrigerator that need using up, but they are a great prep-ahead food. Just roasting them in garlic and thyme gives them a huge amount of flavour, which can brighten up other dishes and salads in a really simple way. I serve them in pitta with torn mozzarella, stirred through couscous, alongside grilled chicken or halloumi, or just tossed into pasta or salads, warm or cold. Once you have roasted them, you can keep them in a sealed container in the refrigerator for up to a week for a quick flavour injection into any meal.

PREP TIME: 5 MINUTES
COOK TIME: 20 MINUTES

500g (1lb 2oz) cherry tomatoes, halved
6 garlic cloves, crushed
1 teaspoon dried thyme
2 teaspoons olive oil
salt and pepper, to taste

1. Preheat the oven to 240°C/220°C fan (475°F), Gas Mark 9. Line a baking tray with nonstick baking paper.

2. In a bowl, mix the cherry tomato halves, garlic, thyme and olive oil and season with salt and pepper.

3. Spread the tomatoes out in a single layer on the prepared tray and roast in the oven for 20 minutes. The tomatoes will be soft, sweet, and caramelized around the edges.

4. Serve hot, or allow to cool, then store in an airtight container in the refrigerator for up to 7 days.

NOTE To save on waste, you can freeze cherry tomatoes if you haven't had a chance to use them or cook them. They do change in texture after being frozen, so aren't great for salads, but will be perfect for cooking into soups, sauces, curries and so on. Simply pop them into a freezer bag or airtight container, label and date them, then store them in the freezer for up to 6 months.

PER SERVING: Calories 61 | Fat 2.7g | Sat Fat 0.4g | Carbs 5.2g | Sugars 4.6g | Fibre 1.6g | Protein 1.7g | Salt 0.26g

CURRIED CHICKPEAS

An absolute breeze to put together, this makes a perfect side dish for another curry, or serve it with rice for a great curry-in-a-hurry main course.

PREP TIME: 2 MINUTES
COOK TIME: 11 MINUTES

spray oil

2 tablespoons tomato purée

1 tablespoon mild curry powder

1 teaspoon ground ginger

1 teaspoon mustard seeds

150ml (¼ pint) vegetable stock

400g (14oz) can of chickpeas, rinsed and drained

400g (14oz) can of green lentils, rinsed and drained

juice of ½ lemon

¼ teaspoon salt

2 large handfuls of baby spinach

TO SERVE

handful of coriander leaves

red chilli, finely chopped

1. Spray a sauté pan with oil, place over a high heat and add the tomato purée, curry powder, ground ginger and mustard seeds. Stir-fry them together for 30 seconds.
2. Pour in the stock, reduce the heat to medium and stir in the chickpeas, lentils, lemon juice and salt. Lower the heat and allow to simmer for 8 minutes, stirring occasionally.
3. Stir in the spinach and leave to simmer for 2 minutes, allowing the leaves to wilt. The consistency should not be liquidy, so if it looks too wet give it a couple of minutes bubbling over a really high heat, constantly stirring, to allow it to thicken up.
4. Serve scattered with coriander and red chilli.

NOTE Powdered vegetable stock (bouillon) is a really useful ingredient to have in your store cupboard for recipes like this that only require a small amount of stock: you can make up exactly what you need without any waste.

PER SERVING: Calories 336 | Fat 5.6g | Sat Fat 0.5g | Carbs 43g | Sugars 4.9g | Fibre 14g | Protein 20g | Salt 1.7g

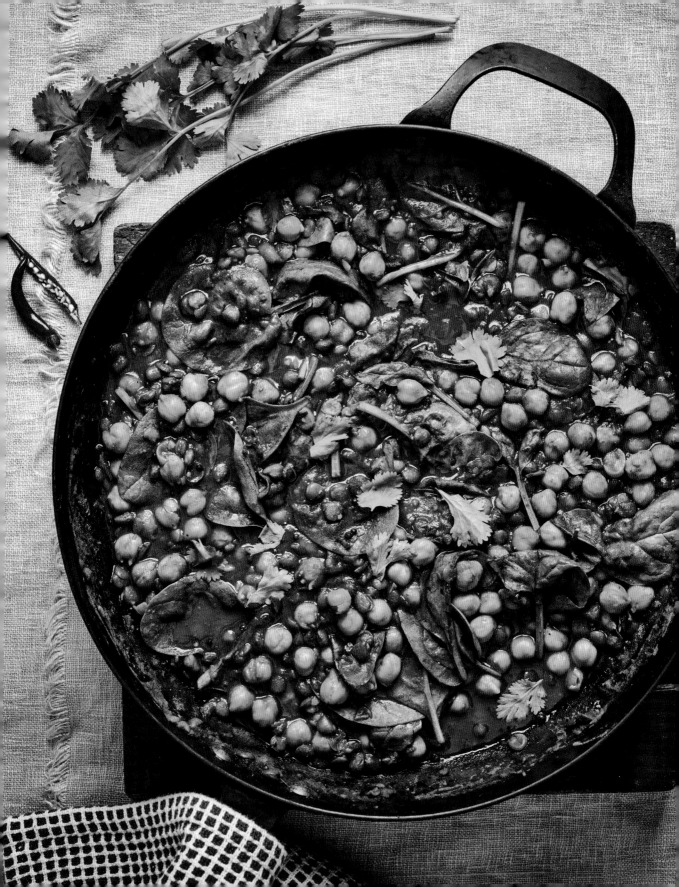

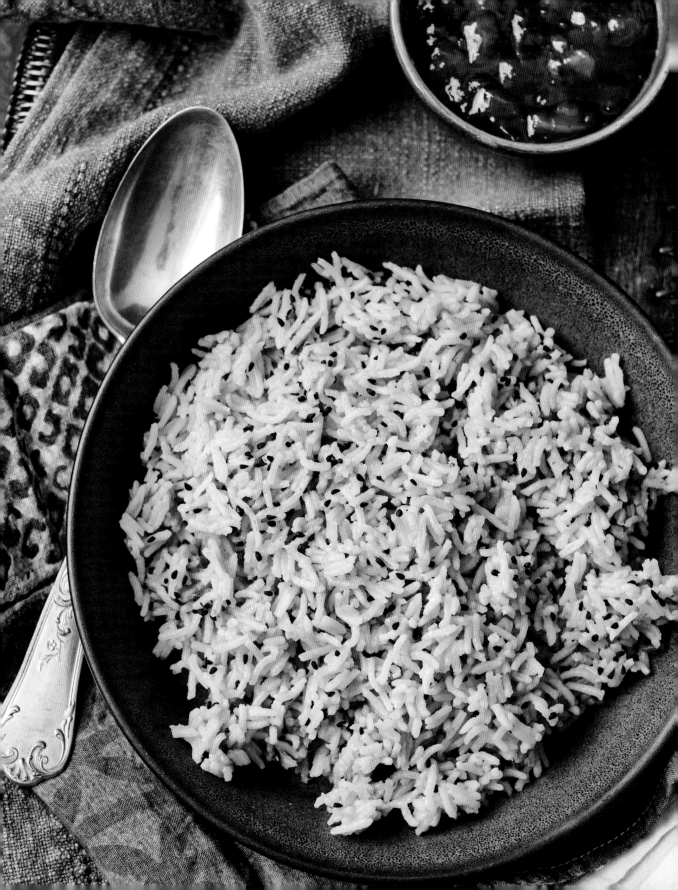

TURMERIC RICE

This richly coloured and flavoursome rice makes a great side dish to any curry and is ideal when you want something a bit more interesting than plain rice, but that doesn't take a lot of extra effort to cook. This also works well alongside salmon or my Brisk Butter Chicken (see page 152).

PREP TIME: 5 MINUTES
COOK TIME: 17 MINUTES

200g (7oz) white basmati rice
2 teaspoons nigella seeds
1 teaspoon ground turmeric
½ teaspoon garlic granules
½ teaspoon onion granules
550ml (1 pint) vegetable stock
½ teaspoon salt
coriander leaves, to serve
   (optional)

1. Rinse the rice thoroughly under cold water, then drain and tip into a saucepan.
2. Mix in the nigella seeds, turmeric and garlic and onion granules, then pour in the stock.
3. Bring to the boil, then reduce the heat to a gentle simmer, place a lid on the pan and simmer gently for 15 minutes.
4. Remove the lid, fluff the rice through with a fork and check it is cooked, then stir through the salt and serve, scattered with coriander, if you like.

NOTE You can make this spicy by adding ½ teaspoon hot chilli powder at the same time as the turmeric.

PER SERVING: Calories 197 | Fat 0.7g | Sat Fat 0.1g | Carbs 42g | Sugars 2g | Fibre 1.6g | Protein 5g | Salt 1.5g

MINI PESHWARI NAANS

I love to have a naan alongside a curry, so here is a super-easy option for an absolutely delicious and simple naan that will outdo anything you can buy in a supermarket, but is hassle-free to make. These are small and are meant as a tasty accompaniment, rather than to fill you up.

PREP TIME: 15 MINUTES
COOK TIME: 12–16 MINUTES

15g (½oz) raisins
12g (¼oz) desiccated coconut
12g (¼oz) flaked almonds
100g (3½oz) fat-free Greek
    yogurt
100g (3½oz) self-raising flour,
    plus extra for dusting
1 teaspoon unsalted butter
salt, to taste

1. In a mini chopper, blend the raisins, coconut and almonds until they are as finely chopped as you can get them.

2. In a large bowl, use a spatula to fold the yogurt into the flour, add a large pinch of salt and keep folding and pressing down until fairly well combined. Next, go in with your hands to thoroughly mix and form the dough into a ball.

3. Divide the ball into 4. Sprinkle a little flour on a work surface and use your hand to push down each piece of dough and shape it into an oval. Keep flattening it, flipping it over and sprinkling on a little extra flour if it gets sticky, until it's about 12cm (4½ inches) long.

4. Take one-quarter of the filling and place it into the middle of a dough oval. Fold the dough over, covering the filling and pressing around the edges to seal it in. Now start again flattening and flipping the dough with your palm to shape the naan. It doesn't matter if a little bit of the filling sneaks out and gets pressed back into the dough, this speckling looks nice when you fry the breads. The final naan should be about 12cm (4½ inches) long and 6cm (2½ inches) wide. Repeat with the remaining dough and filling.

5. Melt the butter in a frying pan and brush it around with a silicone brush to coat the bottom.

6. Place the naans in the pan, 2 at a time, and fry gently for 3–4 minutes on each side. They should be golden-brown on the outside and cooked through in the middle. As long as they are not burning, you can give them an extra 2 minutes if you aren't sure that they are cooked through.

PER NAAN: Calories 169 | Fat 5.8g | Sat Fat 3g | Carbs 22g | Sugars 4g | Fibre 2g | Protein 6.1g | Salt 0.49g

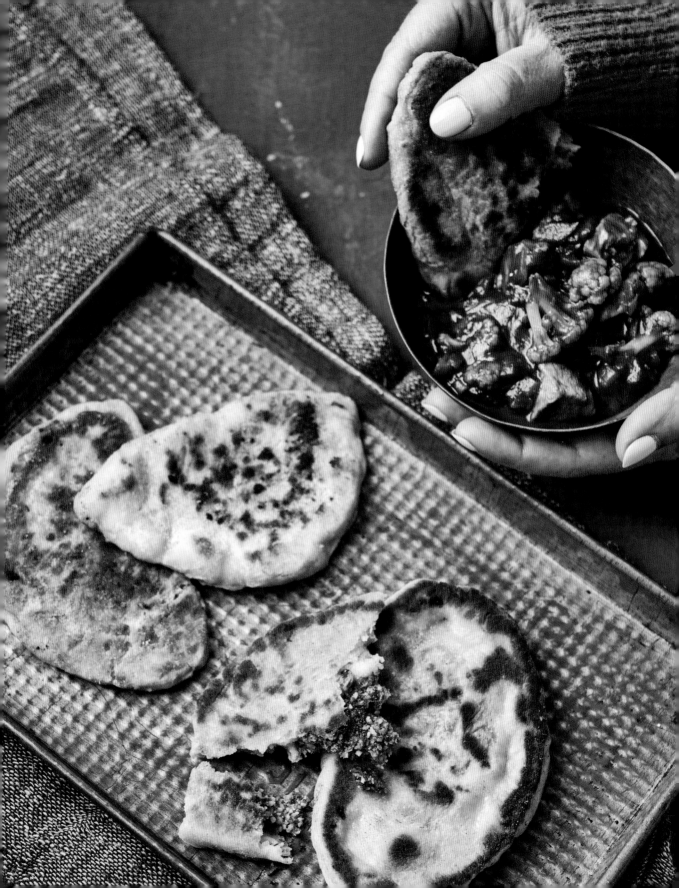

CHAPTER 8

SWEET TOOTH

RASPBERRY MARSHMALLOW PUDDING

This indulgent-tasting dessert has intense raspberry flavour in a sweet and creamy marshmallow base. This is a great recipe to whip up at short notice, as it doesn't require hours in the refrigerator after making it. I serve these in small drinking glasses.

PREP TIME: 2 MINUTES, PLUS 10 MINUTES COOLING
COOK TIME: 5 MINUTES

75g (2¾oz) mini marshmallows
75g (2¾oz) frozen raspberries, plus 50g (1¾oz) extra to serve
75g (2¾oz) fat-free Greek yogurt
25g (1oz) mascarpone cheese
1 teaspoon vanilla extract

1. In small saucepan, heat the marshmallows and the 75g (2¾oz) frozen raspberries for 5 minutes, stirring constantly, by which time the marshmallows should have melted.
2. Remove from the heat and use a spatula to scrape the mixture into a bowl. Leave to cool for 10 minutes, stirring it occasionally to help it lose heat.
3. Stir the yogurt, mascarpone and vanilla through the marshmallow mixture until it is a creamy consistency with no lumps.
4. Place the 50g (1¾oz) frozen raspberries in a plastic bag and bash with a rolling pin until broken down into pieces. Stir the broken-down raspberries through the mixture and scoop into glasses.
5. Serve immediately, or cover and place in the refrigerator until you need them.

HOW TO USE UP LEFTOVER MASCARPONE
Try stirring a spoonful through risotto, orzotto or soup for a creamy finish. Add garlic and herbs and stuff into chicken breasts before baking. Spoon small dollops on to homemade pizza before baking, or simply spread on a bagel and serve with smoked salmon, or add to cooked potatoes before mashing for creamy mash.

PER SERVING: Calories 120 | Fat 2.8g | Sat Fat 1.9g | Carbs 17g | Sugars 14g | Fibre 1.3g | Protein 4.5g | Salt trace

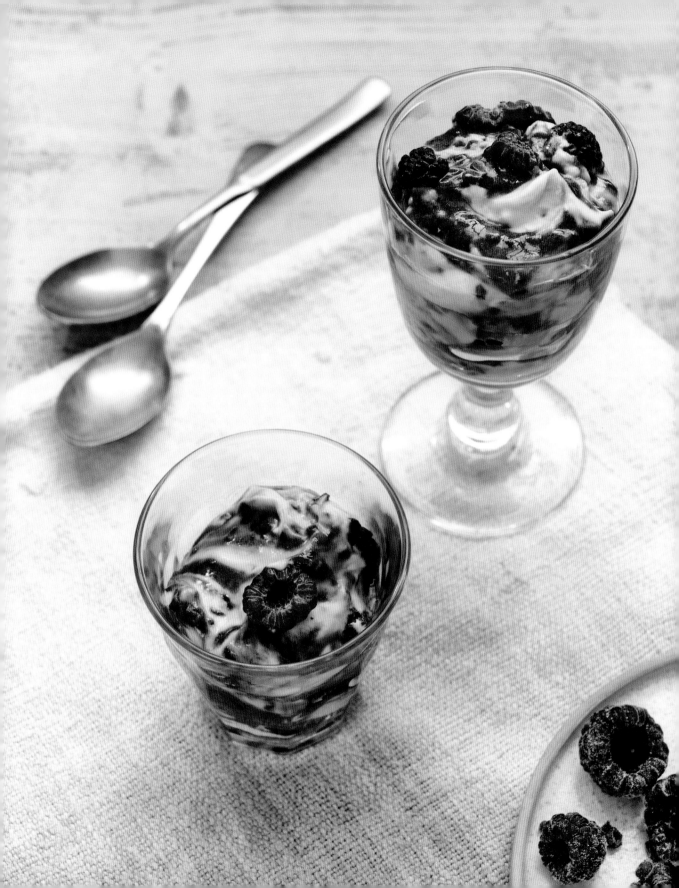

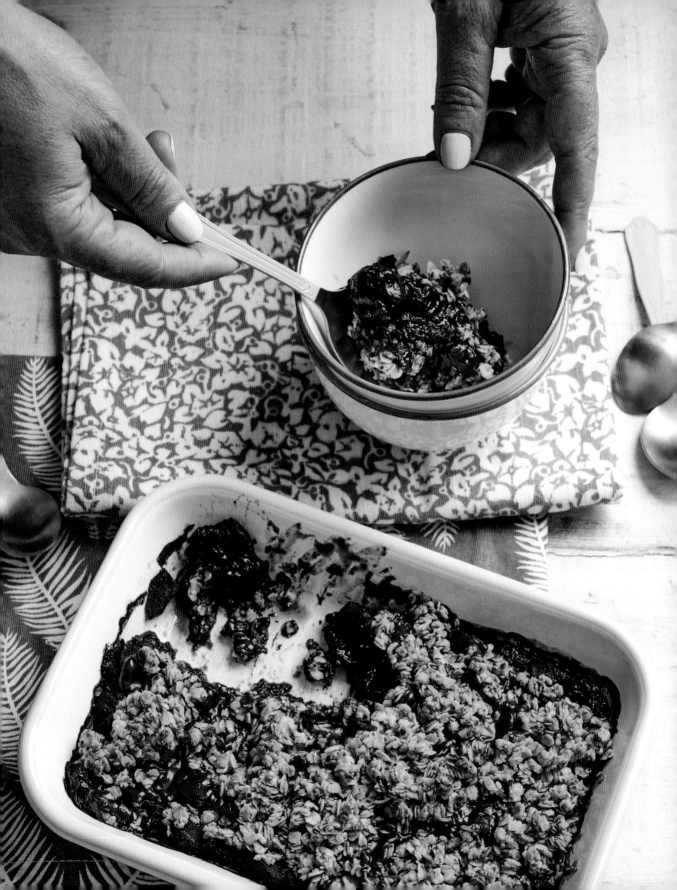

CHERRY CHOCOLATE CRISP

Soft, stewed cherries, apple and vanilla topped with a crumble-like topping with buttery maple oats, dark chocolate and a touch of cinnamon. Frozen cherries that are already pitted are the key to this indulgent-tasting dessert. Eat on its own, or with my quick Funfetti Vanilla Custard (see page 223).

PREP TIME: 5 MINUTES
COOK TIME: 18 MINUTES

1 cooking apple (about 150g / 5½oz), peeled, cored and chopped

250g (9oz) frozen pitted sweet cherries

1 teaspoon vanilla extract

50ml (1¾fl oz) boiling water

2 tablespoons pure maple syrup

1 tablespoon melted unsalted butter

80g (2¾oz) porridge oats

50g (1¾oz) dark chocolate (70 per cent cocoa solids), finely chopped

pinch of ground cinnamon

pinch of salt

1. Preheat the oven to 220°C/200°C fan (425°F), Gas Mark 7.
2. Put the apple, cherries, vanilla and measured boiling water into a small saucepan and simmer for 10 minutes until the apples and cherries are soft. Stir and smash them together while they cook.
3. Meanwhile, in a small bowl, mix together the maple syrup and melted butter. Stir this mixture into the oats in a bowl and add a pinch of salt. Stir the dark chocolate through.
4. Put the cherry mixture into a small baking dish (I use a 20cm/8 inch enamel pie dish), then top with the oats. Sprinkle over the cinnamon.
5. Place into the oven and bake for 8 minutes or until the oats are golden brown. Serve.

A SWEET ALTERNATIVE

When I need added sweetness in a dessert, I will often use maple syrup rather than sugar. In a dessert such as this, the maple flavour enhances the other flavours. Just make sure that you pick up pure maple syrup, rather than maple-flavoured syrup. Although maple syrup is still a free sugar, and therefore needs to be limited in the same way as regular sugar, it does also contain some beneficial minerals.

PER SERVING: Calories 249 | Fat 10g | Sat Fat 5.4g | Carbs 32g | Sugars 17g | Fibre 4.2g | Protein 4.2g | Salt 0.2g

SUMMER FRUITS FRYING PAN SOUFFLÉ

This is a fantastic way to have a really satisfying dessert that is low in calories but can hit the spot and feel like a real treat. Soufflés have a fluffy and airy consistency. I have said this serves one, but it could easily stretch to two if you'd like to share! You can play with the flavours in this; for the compote, try blueberries or blackcurrants, or drizzle some melted peanut butter over a raspberry compote for a PB & J flavour. You could also swap the vanilla for finely grated lemon zest or orange zest, or keep the vanilla flavour and melt some chocolate spread for a chocolate sauce, adding a few toasted hazelnuts.

PREP TIME: 5 MINUTES

COOK TIME: 10 MINUTES

3 eggs, separated (see note on
　page 221)
1 tablespoon caster sugar
1 teaspoon vanilla extract
spray oil or low-calorie cooking
　spray
icing sugar, to serve

**FOR THE SUMMER FRUIT
　COMPOTE**
50g (1¾oz) frozen summer fruits
1 teaspoon honey
2 teaspoons water

1. To make the compote, put the fruit, honey and measured water in a small saucepan and place over a medium heat for 2 minutes, stirring all the time and breaking the fruit down to form a compote. Set aside.

2. In a medium-large bowl, whisk the egg whites with the caster sugar until they are stiff and hold their shape. By hand this should take about 3 minutes, but if you have an electric whisk, it will be much quicker.

3. In a small bowl, use a fork to beat the vanilla extract into the egg yolks.

4. Once the egg whites are stiff, use a wooden spoon to fold the egg yolks into the egg whites gently and carefully: you want to mix them right through the whites without knocking all the air out.

5. Take a nonstick pancake pan or frying pan with a flameproof handle (I use a 20cm/8 inch pan for this) and spray it with spray oil or low-calorie cooking spray. Place over a low heat to start to get the pan warm.

CONTINUED OVERLEAF

PER SERVING: Calories 354 | Fat 16g | Sat Fat 4.5g | Carbs 26g | Sugars 23g | Fibre 2.6g | Protein 22g | Salt 0.68g

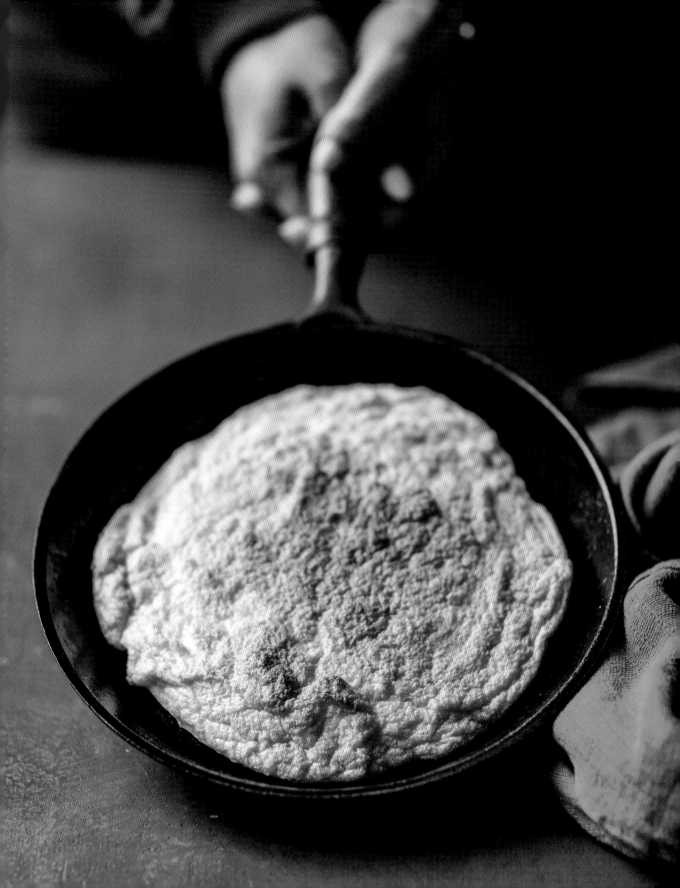

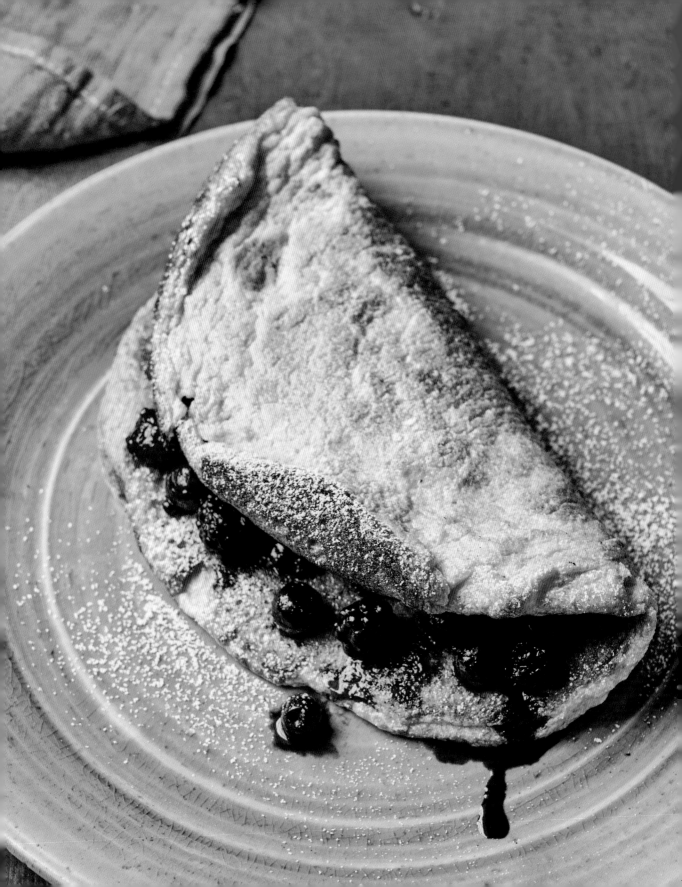

6. Use a spatula to scrape the soufflé mixture into the frying pan, making sure it covers the base, and cook over a low heat for 6 minutes. The aim is to gently toast the bottom and start to cook through the soufflé without burning it. Meanwhile, preheat the grill to medium.

7. After 6 minutes on the hob, place the soufflé pan under the grill and let the top cook for 2 minutes. By this time it should be a light golden brown on top (keep an eye on it to catch it if it starts to burn). Give it a jiggle: it should be a bit jiggly but not sloppy.

8. Use a spatula to carefully loosen underneath the soufflé. I then put a dinner plate on top of the frying pan and flip it upside down to get the soufflé out (be careful not to touch the hot pan!) but you can just use the spatula to carefully lift it out on to a plate.

9. When the soufflé is on the plate, spoon the compote over half of it and fold the other half over the compote. Dust with icing sugar and serve immediately.

HOW TO SEPARATE EGGS
Have 2 bowls ready: you will work over the bowl that will contain the whites. Crack the egg on the edge of the bowl, aiming to crack it at its thickest point (in the middle). Use your thumbs to gently pull apart the 2 halves, holding them carefully, like little cups, to keep the contents in. Carefully tip the yolk from one half to the other at a slight angle, allowing the white to fall into the bowl. Be careful not to break the egg yolk. Keep going until most of the white has dripped out, then drop the yolk into the other bowl.

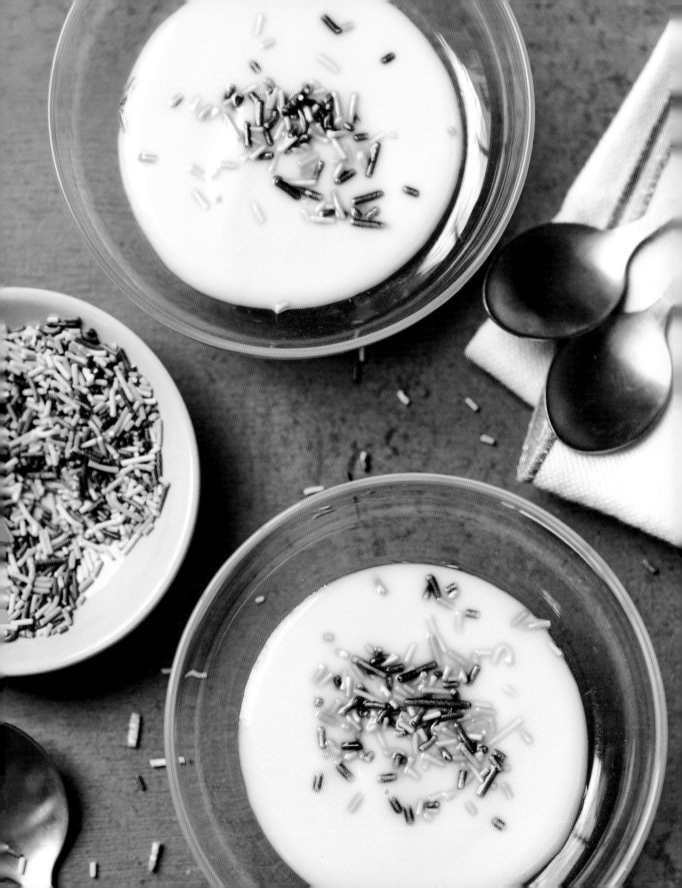

FUNFETTI VANILLA CUSTARD

One of my dad's pet peeves when my brother and I were children was that we loved sprinkling hundreds and thousands over our hot custard, swirling them around to make rainbows. It's so satisfying! So this is childhood comfort food for me. Homemade custard is so quick and easy to make and tastes so much better than the powdered stuff! Most custard recipes use just egg yolks, but I use the whole egg here to save unnecessary faffing. It just means that the custard is a pale cream colour rather than a 'custard yellow', but it still tastes delicious and works perfectly with coloured sugar strands for a fun dessert.

PREP TIME: 2 MINUTES
COOK TIME: 4 MINUTES

200ml (7fl oz) semi-skimmed milk
1 tablespoon cornflour
2 teaspoons sugar
1 egg
½ teaspoon vanilla extract
1 tablespoon rainbow-coloured
    sugar strand sprinkles

1. Set aside a tablespoon of the milk in a small bowl, then pour the rest of the milk into a small saucepan.
2. Mix the cornflour with the reserved milk in the bowl to form a smooth liquid, then add it to the saucepan.
3. Use a fork to whisk in the sugar, egg and vanilla extract.
4. Place the pan over a medium heat and stir it constantly as it heats through. Bring to the boil, then reduce the heat slightly, stirring all the time until it thickens (this will just take a few minutes).
5. Serve in bowls and sprinkle with sugar strands.

NOTE To make chocolate custard, add 25g (1oz) grated dark chocolate (70 per cent cocoa solids) to the ingredients before heating through.

PER SERVING: Calories 168 | Fat 4.5g | Sat Fat 1.9g | Carbs 24g | Sugars 15g | Fibre 0g | Protein 7g | Salt 0.22g

ORANGE & LEMON SPONGE

A simple citrus sponge with a very light orange glaze. Cakes made with yogurt tend to have a slightly chewier texture than traditional sponges, but this can be satisfying and enjoyable in itself. My chief taste-testers love this cake as an after-school snack!

PREP TIME: 7 MINUTES

COOK TIME: 15–20 MINUTES

150g (5½oz) fat-free Greek yogurt
2 eggs
75g (2¾oz) caster sugar
finely grated zest of 1 lemon
finely grated zest of 1 orange
150g (5½oz) self-raising flour
2 tablespoons icing sugar
1 tablespoon orange juice

1. Preheat the oven to 210°C/190°C fan (410°F), Gas Mark 6½. Line a round 20cm (8 inch) diameter shallow cake tin with nonstick baking paper.

2. Put the yogurt in a mixing bowl and add the eggs, caster sugar and zests, then use a fork to thoroughly mix together. Stir in the flour to make a smooth batter.

3. Use a spatula to scrape the mixture into the prepared tin and spread it out evenly. Place on the middle shelf of the oven and bake for 15 minutes.

4. Remove from the oven and test for doneness (see note). If it is not quite cooked in the middle, pop back in the oven for a further 5 minutes.

5. While the cake is cooking, make a simple glaze by mixing the icing sugar with the orange juice.

6. Use a fork to prick some holes in the top of the cake, then use a teaspoon to spread the glaze over the top.

7. Remove from the tin and divide into 8 slices.

NOTE Cakes are notoriously unpredictable and just the smallest differences can change the cooking time, so it's always sensible to check a cake at its thickest part to see if it is fully cooked. First, the cake should feel springy when you (carefully) press your finger on to the top of it. You can use a metal skewer or a sharp knife and slowly insert it into the thickest part of the cake, then slowly pull it out again. If it comes out clean then it is likely that the cake is done; if it comes out streaked with batter, you need to bake the cake for a little longer.

PER SLICE: Calories 147 | Fat 1.7g | Sat Fat 0.4g | Carbs 27g | Sugars 13g | Fibre 0.9g | Protein 5.8g | Salt 0.22g

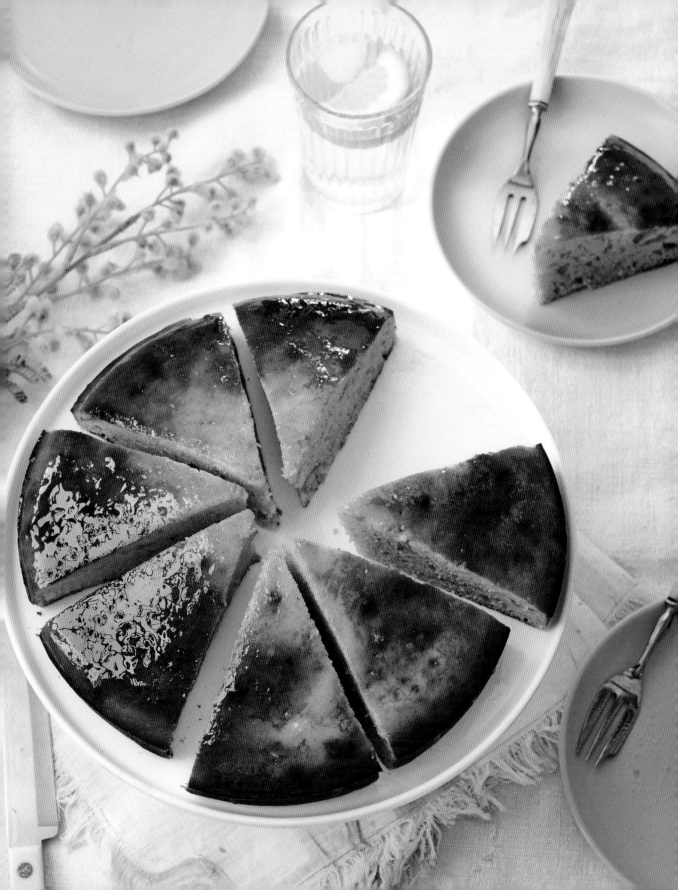

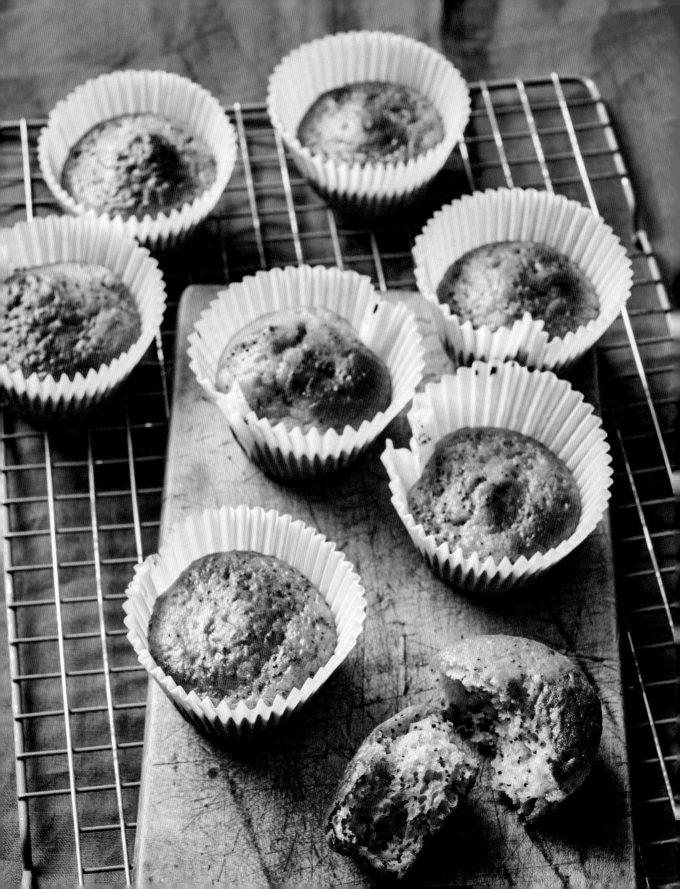

LEMON, HONEY & POPPY SEED BUNS

The classic combination of lemon and poppy seeds is sweetened with honey in these satisfying little buns, a great treat to bake with kids, make for a coffee morning or just for a little sweet pick-me-up. You will need to use nonstick bun cases or a good nonstick muffin tray, as the low fat content means they can be prone to sticking. It's best to let them cool for 5–10 minutes before removing from the case or tray, which should mean they don't stick.

PREP TIME: 5 MINUTES

COOK TIME: 12 MINUTES

100g (3½oz) fat-free Greek yogurt
1 egg
100g (3½oz) honey
1 teaspoon vanilla extract
1 teaspoon olive oil
100g (3½oz) self-raising flour
1 teaspoon baking powder
finely grated zest of 1 lemon
1 tablespoon poppy seeds

1. Preheat the oven to 200°C/180°C fan (400°F), Gas Mark 6. Use a nonstick muffin tray, or line a bun tray with nonstick cake cases.

2. Mix the yogurt, egg, honey, vanilla and oil together in a mixing bowl.

3. Add the flour, baking powder, lemon zest and poppy seeds, then use a wooden spoon to mix everything together into a batter.

4. Spoon about a dessertspoon of mixture into each muffin mould, or cake case, to make 12 buns.

5. Place on the middle tray of the oven and bake for 12 minutes.

6. Allow to cool for 5–10 minutes before removing from the tray or cases.

NOTE If you're making these with kids, or fancy sweetening them up a little more, you could add white chocolate chips to the batter, or make a quick lemon icing from 2 tablespoons icing sugar mixed with 1 tablespoon lemon juice.

PER BUN: Calories 78 | Fat 1.2g | Sat Fat 0.3g | Carbs 13g | Sugars 6.8g | Fibre 0.5g | Protein 3.2g | Salt 0.2g

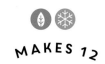

SECRET SWEET POTATO & OAT COOKIES

I call these 'secret' cookies, because you would never know they contained sweet potato unless someone told you, which makes them a perfect healthier snack for fussy kids. I use the term 'healthier', because they do still contain syrup, butter and chocolate chips for a great taste, but I have largely cut down these ingredients and focused on adding fibre with oats, wholemeal flour and sweet potato. So these can be enjoyed as a treat that isn't overly indulgent, but still tastes good.

PREP TIME: 8 MINUTES
COOK TIME: 12 MINUTES

75g (2¾oz) porridge oats
75g (2¾oz) wholemeal flour
1 teaspoon baking powder
1 teaspoon ground cinnamon
¼ teaspoon salt
25g (1oz) milk or dark chocolate chips
75g (2¾oz) grated sweet potato
1 teaspoon vanilla extract
3 tablespoons golden syrup (45g/1½oz)
1 egg
25g (1oz) melted unsalted butter

1. Preheat the oven to 200°C/180°C fan (400°F), Gas Mark 6. Line a large baking tray with nonstick baking paper.
2. Put all the dry ingredients in a large bowl with the sweet potato, then add the wet ingredients and use a wooden spoon to thoroughly combine everything together.
3. Use the mixture to make 12 balls, each about the size of a golf ball, laying them out on the prepared tray as you make them.
4. Use a fork to gently press down on top of each cookie to slightly flatten it and leave an imprint.
5. Bake for 12 minutes in the oven; they should be a lovely golden-brown colour. If they look a bit pale, you can bake them for an extra couple of minutes.

NOTE These are best served warm, fresh from the oven, but you can store them in an airtight container for up to 3 days (allow them to thoroughly cool first), or you can freeze them. If you are having them from the freezer, allow them to defrost and then pop them into an oven preheated to 200°C/180°C fan (400°F), Gas Mark 6 for 5 minutes, to refresh and slightly crisp them up again.

PER COOKIE: Calories 103 | Fat 3.4g | Sat Fat 1.7g | Carbs 15g | Sugars 5.8g | Fibre 1.4g | Protein 2.3g | Salt 0.32g

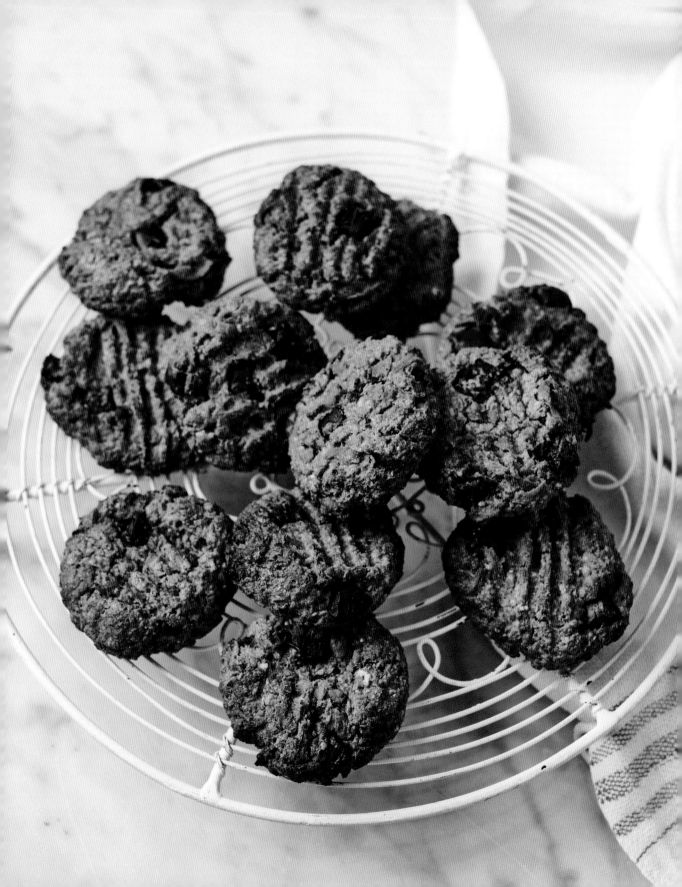

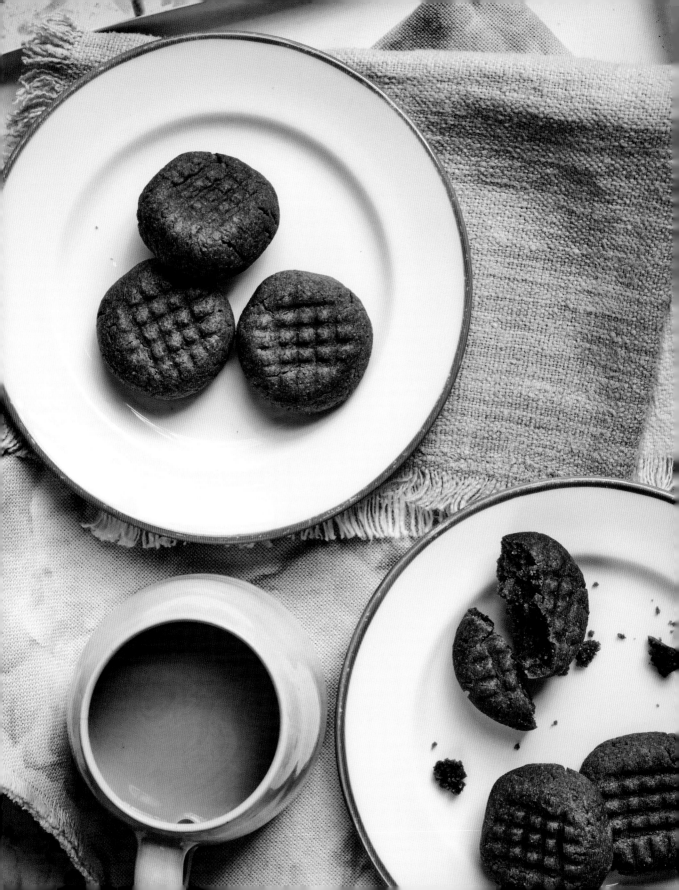

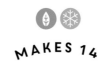

THE SIMPLEST PEANUT BUTTER COOKIES

These are not a low-calorie option, but honestly, I think that there's no harm in having a treat every now and again. Just make sure it is an enjoyable indulgence: making something delicious yourself is so much more satisfying than wasting calories on bought snacks which often don't taste as good! These are just brilliant to cook with kids, or as a super-quick recipe to whip up if you have unexpected visitors arriving. I'm not sure there is a quicker homemade cookie out there!

PREP TIME: 2 MINUTES
COOK TIME: 8 MINUTES

200g (7oz) smooth peanut butter
100g (3½oz) soft dark brown sugar
1 egg
1 teaspoon vanilla extract
pinch of salt

1. Preheat the oven to 200°C/180°C fan (400°F), Gas Mark 6. Line a large baking tray with nonstick baking paper.
2. In a bowl, combine the peanut butter, sugar, egg, vanilla and salt into a smooth batter.
3. Use your hands to roll it into 14 walnut-sized balls, spacing them out over the prepared tray (you can use 2 teaspoons if you prefer not to get your hands messy, but the cookies won't be as neat).
4. Use a fork to press down firmly on top of each cookie, first one way, then the other, to create a cross-hatch pattern on top. (I find that having a mug of water next to me, and dipping the fork in while I'm doing this, prevents it from sticking to the cookies.)
5. Bake for 8 minutes; they should be golden brown – just keep an eye on them as they can catch and burn very quickly.
6. The cookies will be very soft when they first come out of the oven, so allow them to cool for 10 minutes or so before gently removing them from the baking paper.

NOTE You can add ½ teaspoon ground cinnamon, some chocolate chips or some crushed peanuts to the cookie dough if you want to jazz these up a bit.

PER COOKIE: Calories 124 | Fat 7.8g | Sat Fat 1.9g | Carbs 8.7g | Sugars 7.8g | Fibre 0.9g | Protein 4.2g | Salt 0.18g

RECIPE LIST

INDEX

UK-US GLOSSARY

UK	US	UK	US
aubergine	eggplant	semi-skimmed milk	reduced-fat milk
bacon medallions	fat-free bacon		/ 2% milk
	rounds	single cream	half and half
borlotti beans	cranberry beans	sirloin steak	porterhouse steak
Bird's eye chilli	Thai chilli	spring onions	scallions
casserole dish	Dutch oven	streaky bacon rashers	regular American
caster sugar	superfine sugar		bacon slices
cheese toastie	grilled cheese	tenderstem broccoli	broccolini
chestnut mushrooms	cremini	tin (cake, roasting)	pan
	mushrooms	wholemeal	whole wheat
chilli flakes	red pepper flakes		
cold-water prawn	Northern prawn		
coriander	cilantro		
cornflour	corn starch		
courgette	zucchini		
cress	baby mustard		
	sprouts		
custard	crème anglaise		
dark chocolate	bittersweet chocolate		
dessicated coconut	shredded coconut		
flaked almonds	sliced almonds		
frying pan	skillet		
grill	broil		
golden syrup	light corn syrup		
icing sugar	confectioner's		
	sugar		
king prawns	jumbo shrimp		
kitchen paper	paper towels		
minced meat	ground meat		
muffins	English muffins		
plain flour	all-purpose flour		
prawns	shrimp		
red pepper	red bell pepper		
rump steak	sirloin steak/scotch fillet		
self-raising flour	self-rising flour		

ACKNOWLEDGEMENTS

Thank you to my family. My husband, Darren, and my lovely daughters, Miette and Marlie. They are the reason behind my determination to work as hard as I can to make The Slimming Foodie a success, and give me many moments of joy and happiness which help to balance out the exhaustion and self-doubt which I have discovered are a part of the process for every book I write! A hug from any one of them always makes everything feel better. Also to Darren for doing so much in the background for The Slimming Foodie. Thanks to my Mum and Dad, who are always happy to help out, I am so lucky to have you both.

To my amazing friends. My little neighbourhood gang, who are always there for dog walks, tea, prosecco and natters: I'm so happy to have you all on my doorstep. Special thanks to Sarah T and Maria, for helping out as admins on my ever-growing Facebook group: I am so grateful that, alongside their busy jobs and families, they are willing to help out on that ever-consuming task. Again to Sarah T, and to my lovely friend Lorraine, for helping me to brainstorm recipe ideas. To Shaz and Han, for providing podcast-length voice notes to keep me in touch when I'm in full book-writing mode, and providing me with plenty of giggles along the way.

To my agent, Heather Holden-Brown, for her guidance and understanding of the way that I work. Thank you to my editor, Natalie Bradley, for being just generally fantastic, fun, insightful and available.

Thank you to Lucy Bannell, for helping to get my manuscript into shape and pick up on details that I've missed. To Sybella Stephens for overseeing the whole process from start to finish, and to the many team members at Octopus who I haven't met yet, but I know are there behind the scenes to bring the book to life. To Karen Baker and Hazel O'Brien for all their work on publicity and marketing, and Kevin Hawkins and Marianne Laidlaw for everything they do on the sales side. To Yasia Williams and her team of designers for making the books look beautiful and colourful. And to everyone at Octopus who hasn't had a personal mention but make up a brilliant team.

Thank you to my amazing shoot team. Chris Terry for the stunning photography which is so integral to the feel of the book. To Henrietta Clancy, food stylist, who works so hard to get through the recipes every day and manages to make each and every one look beautiful and appetising. To Tamsin Weston, prop stylist, for always hitting the nail on the head when choosing just the right linens, backgrounds, dishes, pans and cutlery. All the team are just absolutely lovely, professional and talented, but still such fun to work with and I'm so pleased that they have now worked on all three of my books.

The biggest thanks to everyone who has supported The Slimming Foodie online and bought my first two books. It's been lovely to see so many of the recipes being enjoyed and I'm so pleased to have such a positive community to share photos and advice. Seeing the recipes come to life in Instagram and Facebook is always a highlight of a new book being released, and I really appreciate the kind comments, messages and reviews.